Food & Fitness
JOURNAL

STAY ON TRACK & ACHIEVE YOUR GOALS

STERLING
New York

STERLING
New York

An Imprint of Sterling Publishing Co., Inc.
1166 Avenue of the Americas
New York, NY 10036

ISBN 978-1-4549-3233-8

Distributed in Canada by Sterling Publishing Co., Inc.
c/o Canadian Manda Group, 664 Annette Street
Toronto, Ontario, M6S 2C8, Canada
Distributed in the United Kingdom by GMC Distribution Services
Castle Place, 166 High Street, Lewes, East Sussex, BN7 1XU, United Kingdom
Distributed in Australia by NewSouth Books
45 Beach Street, Coogee, NSW 2034, Australia

For information about custom editions, special sales,
and premium and corporate purchases, please contact
Sterling Special Sales at 800-805-5489
or specialsales@sterlingpublishing.com.

Manufactured in Canada

2 4 6 8 10 9 7 5 3 1

sterlingpublishing.com

Cover design by Igor Satanovsky
Picture Credit: ©fonikum/iStock

Contents

Introduction

U se this journal to record your daily food intake and exercise. It will show you your favorite foods and fitness activities, what you can't resist, and what you need to cut from or add to your health routine. In the notes section, comment on how you're feeling that day, where you went right or wrong, foods or exercises that you want to try, or something that inspired you to stay on course.

To maintain your current weight, you have to consume about 12 to 15 calories per day for every pound you weigh. If you weigh 175 pounds, you need to eat 2,100 to 2,625 calories per day to stay there. To lose weight, you have to eat fewer calories. To gain weight, you need to eat more. Women should eat at least 1,200 calories per day, and men should eat at least 1,500 to maintain a healthy diet.

Protein, fats, and carbohydrates are three of the most important energy-producing nutrients for the human body, but don't overdo or exclude any of them. Getting your daily protein requirements from lean meats, cheese, yogurt, and eggs is smart because each of those foods has high levels of protein and additional nutritional value. Make sure you're getting all of the recommended vitamins and minerals and not eating "empty" calories—foods with little nutritional value that are high in carbs and fat. Eat as little saturated fat as possible.

To figure out your recommended caloric intake and daily balance of protein, fats, and carbs, use the formulas and tables that follow this introduction. At the back of this journal is a list of common foods and their nutrient contents, which will help you keep track of your daily food intake when eating out or when your food doesn't have a nutritional label. Also included are lists of foods recommended for essential minerals and vitamins.

Drink plenty of water. It speeds various metabolic processes, moves waste from your body, and helps you shed stored fat. Like oil in an engine, water keeps your body moving.

Daily exercise will strengthen your muscles, heart, and lungs, give you more energy, and help you lose or gain weight. At the back of this journal is a comprehensive table showing how many calories per hour a variety of exercises burns.

To achieve your goals, it's important to set the right ones and then write them down. When you set a particular goal, list why you're setting it. Write down everything you want to happen as a result of reaching your target result. Everyone wants to look better, but *why* do you want to look better? Is it to have more confidence, energy, or strength? What does that mean for you? Be specific and detailed. Is it to be able to enjoy your life and family when older? How does that look in your mind? Set goals that focus on the process—how you plan to reach them and the effort you put toward them—rather than just the outcome.

If your goal involves losing weight, note that healthy weight loss averages about two pounds per week. If you're more than 50 pounds overweight, you may see more rapid results in the beginning. To lose weight properly and keep it off, set a healthy and realistic goal.

To set your goals, start by find your daily balances using the formulas below and the tables on the pages that follow.

$$\underline{\hspace{3cm}} \times 13.5 = \underline{\hspace{3cm}}$$

current weight　　current average calorie intake

Daily Calorie Balance

Current average calorie intake　　=　　maintain current weight

Current average calorie intake − 500　=　_____ calories = 1 pound lost per week

Current average calorie intake − 750　=　_____ calories = 1–1½ pounds lost per week

Current average calorie intake − 1,000 = _____ calories = 2 pounds lost per week

If you want a quarter of your daily calories to come from protein, a quarter from fat, and half from carbohydrates—a healthy overall balance—use the formulas below to determine your daily balances of each.

Daily Protein Balance

$$\underline{\hspace{2cm}} \times 0.25 \quad \div \quad 4 \quad = \quad \underline{\hspace{1cm}} \text{ grams}$$
Daily Calorie Balance　　(cals in 1 gram of protein)　　Daily Protein Balance

Daily Fat Balance

$$\underline{\hspace{2cm}} \times 0.25 \quad \div \quad 9 \quad = \quad \underline{\hspace{1cm}} \text{ grams}$$
Daily Calorie Balance　　(cals in 1 gram of fat)　　Daily Fat Balance

Daily Carb Balance

$$\underline{\hspace{2cm}} \times 0.5 \quad \div \quad 4 \quad = \quad \underline{\hspace{1cm}} \text{ grams}$$
Daily Calorie Balance　　(cals in 1 gram of carbs)　　Daily Carbs Balance

If you want a different overall balance of protein, fat, and carbs, adjust the decimal percentages above accordingly. Remember to recalculate your daily balances each week based on your current weight.

Daily Nutritional Goals

Nutrient	Female 19–30	Male 19–30	Female 31–50	Male, 31–50	Female 51+	Male, 51+
Calories	see tables on pages 8-9					
Protein, g	46	56	46	56	46	56
Protein %	10–35	10–35	10–35	10–35	10–35	10–35
Fat %	20–35	20–35	20–35	20–35	20–35	20–35
Carbs, g	130	130	130	130	130	130
Carbs %	45–65	45–65	45–65	45–65	45–65	45–65
Dietary Fiber	28	33.6	25.2	30.8	22.4	28
Calcium, mg	1,000	1,000	1,000	1,000	1,000	1,000
Vitamin D, IU	600	600	600	600	600	600
Iron, mg	18	8	18	8	8	8
Potassium, mg	4,700	4,700	4,700	4,700	4,700	4,700
Sodium, mg	2,300	2,300	2,300	2,300	2,300	2,300

From the USDA Dietary Guidelines for Americans, 2015–2020

Calories Needed per Day by Gender, Age & Activity Level

Females*

Age	Sedentary	Moderately Active	Active
18	1,800	2,000	2,400
19-20	2,000	2,200	2,400
21-25	2,000	2,200	2,400
26-30	1,800	2,000	2,400
31-35	1,800	2,000	2,200
36-40	1,800	2,000	2,200
41-45	1,800	2,000	2,200
46-50	1,800	2,000	2,200
51-55	1,600	1,800	2,200
61-65	1,600	1,800	2,000
66-70	1,600	1,800	2,000
71-75	1,600	1,800	2,000
76+	1,600	1,800	2,000

* Not including women who are pregnant or breastfeeding

Males

Age	Sedentary	Moderately Active	Active
18	2,400	2,800	3,200
19-20	2,600	2,800	3,000
21-25	2,400	2,800	3,000
26-30	2,400	2,600	3,000
31-35	2,400	2,600	3,000
36-40	2,400	2,600	2,800
41-45	2,200	2,600	2,800
46-50	2,200	2,400	2,800
51-55	2,200	2,400	2,800
61-65	2,000	2,400	2,600
66-70	2,000	2,200	2,600
71-75	2,000	2,200	2,600
76+	2,000	2,200	2,400

From the USDA Dietary Guidelines for Americans, 2015–2020

GOAL SHEETS

GOAL

_____

_____

_____

_____

_____

_____

REASONS

_____

_____

_____

_____

_____

_____

PLAN

_____

_____

_____

_____

_____

_____

_____

DAILY FOOD TARGET

DAILY EXERCISE TARGET

WEEKLY EXERCISE TARGET

STATS

	MEASUREMENTS	BEFORE	AFTER
WEIGHT			
NECK			
UPPER ARMS			
CHEST			
WAIST			
HIPS			
THIGHS			
CALVES			
BLOOD PRESSURE			
CHOLESTEROL			

GOAL SHEETS

GOAL

_____

_____

_____

_____

_____

REASONS

_____

_____

_____

_____

_____

PLAN

_____

_____

_____

_____

_____

_____

DAILY FOOD TARGET

DAILY EXERCISE TARGET

WEEKLY EXERCISE TARGET

STATS

	MEASUREMENTS	BEFORE	AFTER
WEIGHT			
NECK			
UPPER ARMS			
CHEST			
WAIST			
HIPS			
THIGHS			
CALVES			
BLOOD PRESSURE			
CHOLESTEROL			

GOAL SHEETS

GOAL

_____

_____

_____

_____

_____

REASONS

_____

_____

_____

_____

PLAN

_____

_____

_____

_____

_____

_____

DAILY FOOD TARGET

DAILY EXERCISE TARGET

WEEKLY EXERCISE TARGET

STATS

	MEASUREMENTS	BEFORE	AFTER
WEIGHT			
NECK			
UPPER ARMS			
CHEST			
WAIST			
HIPS			
THIGHS			
CALVES			
BLOOD PRESSURE			
CHOLESTEROL			

Weekly Tracker

Track your progress by recording any or all of the statistics below. Use the blanks at the bottom to record any other variables, such as meals eaten out or units of alcohol consumed.

	WEEK 1	WEEK 2	WEEK 3	WEEK 4	WEEK 5
WEIGHT					
NECK					
UPPER ARMS					
CHEST					
WAIST					
HIPS					
THIGHS					
CALVES					
BLOOD PRESSURE					
CHOLESTEROL LEVEL					
AVG DAILY CALORIES					
AVG DAILY FAT					
AVG DAILY PROTEIN					
AVG DAILY CARBS					
AVG DAILY WATER					
AVG DAILY CALORIES BURNED					
AVG DAILY HOURS OF EXERCISE					

	WEEK 6	WEEK 7	WEEK 8	WEEK 9	WEEK 10
WEIGHT					
NECK					
UPPER ARMS					
CHEST					
WAIST					
HIPS					
THIGHS					
CALVES					
BLOOD PRESSURE					
CHOLESTEROL LEVEL					
AVG DAILY CALORIES					
AVG DAILY FAT					
AVG DAILY PROTEIN					
AVG DAILY CARBS					
AVG DAILY WATER					
AVG DAILY CALORIES BURNED					
AVG DAILY HOURS OF EXERCISE					

	WEEK 1	WEEK 2	WEEK 3	WEEK 4	WEEK 5
WEIGHT					
NECK					
UPPER ARMS					
CHEST					
WAIST					
HIPS					
THIGHS					
CALVES					
BLOOD PRESSURE					
CHOLESTEROL LEVEL					
AVG DAILY CALORIES					
AVG DAILY FAT					
AVG DAILY PROTEIN					
AVG DAILY CARBS					
AVG DAILY WATER					
AVG DAILY CALORIES BURNED					
AVG DAILY HOURS OF EXERCISE					

	WEEK 6	WEEK 7	WEEK 8	WEEK 9	WEEK 10
WEIGHT					
NECK					
UPPER ARMS					
CHEST					
WAIST					
HIPS					
THIGHS					
CALVES					
BLOOD PRESSURE					
CHOLESTEROL LEVEL					
AVG DAILY CALORIES					
AVG DAILY FAT					
AVG DAILY PROTEIN					
AVG DAILY CARBS					
AVG DAILY WATER					
AVG DAILY CALORIES BURNED					
AVG DAILY HOURS OF EXERCISE					

FOOD LOG

DATE _____

WEIGHT _____

TIME	AMOUNT	FOOD	CALORIES	PROTEIN	FAT	CARBS	FIBER	SODIUM	
		TOTALS							
		GOALS							

VITAMINS/SUPPLEMENTS

8-ounce glasses of water

EXERCISE LOG

CARDIO				
ACTIVITY	LEVEL	DISTANCE	MINUTES	CALS BURNED

WEIGHTS			
ACTIVITY	WEIGHT	REPS	CALS BURNED

GOAL TRACKER			
ORIGINAL	CURRENT	CHANGE	AMOUNT REMAINING

FOOD LOG

DATE _____

WEIGHT _____

TIME	AMOUNT	FOOD	CALORIES	PROTEIN	FAT	CARBS	FIBER	SODIUM
		TOTALS						
		GOALS						

VITAMINS/SUPPLEMENTS

_____

_____

8-ounce glasses of water

EXERCISE LOG

CARDIO				
ACTIVITY	LEVEL	DISTANCE	MINUTES	CALS BURNED

WEIGHTS			
ACTIVITY	WEIGHT	REPS	CALS BURNED

GOAL TRACKER			
ORIGINAL	CURRENT	CHANGE	AMOUNT REMAINING

FOOD LOG

DATE _____

WEIGHT _____

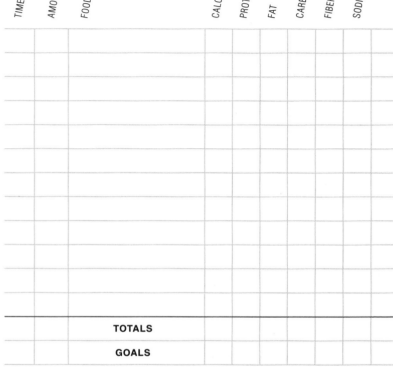

TIME	AMOUNT	FOOD	CALORIES	PROTEIN	FAT	CARBS	FIBER	SODIUM	
		TOTALS							
		GOALS							

VITAMINS/SUPPLEMENTS

8-ounce glasses of water

EXERCISE LOG

CARDIO				
ACTIVITY	LEVEL	DISTANCE	MINUTES	CALS BURNED

WEIGHTS			
ACTIVITY	WEIGHT	REPS	CALS BURNED

GOAL TRACKER			
ORIGINAL	CURRENT	CHANGE	AMOUNT REMAINING

FOOD LOG

DATE _____

WEIGHT _____

TIME	AMOUNT	FOOD	CALORIES	PROTEIN	FAT	CARBS	FIBER	SODIUM
		TOTALS						
		GOALS						

VITAMINS/SUPPLEMENTS

_____

_____

8-ounce glasses of water

EXERCISE LOG

CARDIO				
ACTIVITY	LEVEL	DISTANCE	MINUTES	CALS BURNED

WEIGHTS			
ACTIVITY	WEIGHT	REPS	CALS BURNED

GOAL TRACKER			
ORIGINAL	CURRENT	CHANGE	AMOUNT REMAINING

FOOD LOG

DATE _____

WEIGHT _____

TIME	AMOUNT	FOOD	CALORIES	PROTEIN	FAT	CARBS	FIBER	SODIUM
		TOTALS						
		GOALS						

VITAMINS/SUPPLEMENTS

_____

_____

8-ounce glasses of water

EXERCISE LOG

CARDIO				
ACTIVITY	LEVEL	DISTANCE	MINUTES	CALS BURNED

WEIGHTS			
ACTIVITY	WEIGHT	REPS	CALS BURNED

GOAL TRACKER			
ORIGINAL	CURRENT	CHANGE	AMOUNT REMAINING

FOOD LOG

DATE _____

WEIGHT _____

TIME	AMOUNT	FOOD	CALORIES	PROTEIN	FAT	CARBS	FIBER	SODIUM
		TOTALS						
		GOALS						

VITAMINS/SUPPLEMENTS

_____

_____

8-ounce glasses of water

EXERCISE LOG

CARDIO				
ACTIVITY	LEVEL	DISTANCE	MINUTES	CALS BURNED

WEIGHTS			
ACTIVITY	WEIGHT	REPS	CALS BURNED

GOAL TRACKER			
ORIGINAL	CURRENT	CHANGE	AMOUNT REMAINING

FOOD LOG

DATE _____

WEIGHT _____

TIME	AMOUNT	FOOD	CALORIES	PROTEIN	FAT	CARBS	FIBER	SODIUM
		TOTALS						
		GOALS						

VITAMINS/SUPPLEMENTS

_____

_____

8-ounce glasses of water

EXERCISE LOG

CARDIO

ACTIVITY	LEVEL	DISTANCE	MINUTES	CALS BURNED

WEIGHTS

ACTIVITY	WEIGHT	REPS	CALS BURNED

GOAL TRACKER

ORIGINAL	CURRENT	CHANGE	AMOUNT REMAINING

FOOD LOG

DATE _____

WEIGHT _____

TIME	AMOUNT	FOOD	CALORIES	PROTEIN	FAT	CARBS	FIBER	SODIUM
		TOTALS						
		GOALS						

VITAMINS/SUPPLEMENTS

_____

_____

8-ounce glasses of water

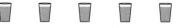

EXERCISE LOG

CARDIO				
ACTIVITY	LEVEL	DISTANCE	MINUTES	CALS BURNED

WEIGHTS			
ACTIVITY	WEIGHT	REPS	CALS BURNED

GOAL TRACKER			
ORIGINAL	CURRENT	CHANGE	AMOUNT REMAINING

FOOD LOG

DATE _____

WEIGHT _____

TIME	AMOUNT	FOOD	CALORIES	PROTEIN	FAT	CARBS	FIBER	SODIUM
		TOTALS						
		GOALS						

VITAMINS/SUPPLEMENTS

_____

_____

8-ounce glasses of water

EXERCISE LOG

CARDIO				
ACTIVITY	LEVEL	DISTANCE	MINUTES	CALS BURNED

WEIGHTS			
ACTIVITY	WEIGHT	REPS	CALS BURNED

GOAL TRACKER			
ORIGINAL	CURRENT	CHANGE	AMOUNT REMAINING

FOOD LOG

DATE _____

WEIGHT _____

TIME	AMOUNT	FOOD	CALORIES	PROTEIN	FAT	CARBS	FIBER	SODIUM	
		TOTALS							
		GOALS							

VITAMINS/SUPPLEMENTS

_____

_____

8-ounce glasses of water

EXERCISE LOG

CARDIO				
ACTIVITY	LEVEL	DISTANCE	MINUTES	CALS BURNED

WEIGHTS			
ACTIVITY	WEIGHT	REPS	CALS BURNED

GOAL TRACKER			
ORIGINAL	CURRENT	CHANGE	AMOUNT REMAINING

FOOD LOG

DATE _____

WEIGHT _____

TIME	AMOUNT	FOOD	CALORIES	PROTEIN	FAT	CARBS	FIBER	SODIUM	
		TOTALS							
		GOALS							

VITAMINS/SUPPLEMENTS

_____

_____

8-ounce glasses of water

EXERCISE LOG

CARDIO

ACTIVITY	LEVEL	DISTANCE	MINUTES	CALS BURNED

WEIGHTS

ACTIVITY	WEIGHT	REPS	CALS BURNED

GOAL TRACKER

ORIGINAL	CURRENT	CHANGE	AMOUNT REMAINING

FOOD LOG

DATE _____

WEIGHT _____

TIME	AMOUNT	FOOD	CALORIES	PROTEIN	FAT	CARBS	FIBER	SODIUM
		TOTALS						
		GOALS						

VITAMINS/SUPPLEMENTS

_____

_____

8-ounce glasses of water

EXERCISE LOG

CARDIO				
ACTIVITY	LEVEL	DISTANCE	MINUTES	CALS BURNED

WEIGHTS			
ACTIVITY	WEIGHT	REPS	CALS BURNED

GOAL TRACKER			
ORIGINAL	CURRENT	CHANGE	AMOUNT REMAINING

FOOD LOG

DATE _____

WEIGHT _____

TIME	AMOUNT	FOOD	CALORIES	PROTEIN	FAT	CARBS	FIBER	SODIUM
		TOTALS						
		GOALS						

VITAMINS/SUPPLEMENTS

_____

_____

8-ounce glasses of water

EXERCISE LOG

CARDIO				
ACTIVITY	LEVEL	DISTANCE	MINUTES	CALS BURNED

WEIGHTS			
ACTIVITY	WEIGHT	REPS	CALS BURNED

GOAL TRACKER			
ORIGINAL	CURRENT	CHANGE	AMOUNT REMAINING

FOOD LOG

DATE _____

WEIGHT _____

TIME	AMOUNT	FOOD	CALORIES	PROTEIN	FAT	CARBS	FIBER	SODIUM
		TOTALS						
		GOALS						

VITAMINS/SUPPLEMENTS

_____

_____

8-ounce glasses of water

EXERCISE LOG

CARDIO				
ACTIVITY	LEVEL	DISTANCE	MINUTES	CALS BURNED

WEIGHTS			
ACTIVITY	WEIGHT	REPS	CALS BURNED

GOAL TRACKER			
ORIGINAL	CURRENT	CHANGE	AMOUNT REMAINING

FOOD LOG

DATE _____

WEIGHT _____

TIME	AMOUNT	FOOD	CALORIES	PROTEIN	FAT	CARBS	FIBER	SODIUM
		TOTALS						
		GOALS						

VITAMINS/SUPPLEMENTS

_____

_____

8-ounce glasses of water

EXERCISE LOG

CARDIO				
ACTIVITY	LEVEL	DISTANCE	MINUTES	CALS BURNED

WEIGHTS			
ACTIVITY	WEIGHT	REPS	CALS BURNED

GOAL TRACKER			
ORIGINAL	CURRENT	CHANGE	AMOUNT REMAINING

FOOD LOG

DATE _____

WEIGHT _____

TIME	AMOUNT	FOOD	CALORIES	PROTEIN	FAT	CARBS	FIBER	SODIUM	
		TOTALS							
		GOALS							

VITAMINS/SUPPLEMENTS

_____

_____

8-ounce glasses of water

EXERCISE LOG

CARDIO				
ACTIVITY	LEVEL	DISTANCE	MINUTES	CALS BURNED

WEIGHTS			
ACTIVITY	WEIGHT	REPS	CALS BURNED

GOAL TRACKER			
ORIGINAL	CURRENT	CHANGE	AMOUNT REMAINING

FOOD LOG

DATE _____

WEIGHT _____

TIME	AMOUNT	FOOD	CALORIES	PROTEIN	FAT	CARBS	FIBER	SODIUM	
		TOTALS							
		GOALS							

VITAMINS/SUPPLEMENTS

_____

_____

8-ounce glasses of water

EXERCISE LOG

CARDIO				
ACTIVITY	LEVEL	DISTANCE	MINUTES	CALS BURNED

WEIGHTS			
ACTIVITY	WEIGHT	REPS	CALS BURNED

GOAL TRACKER			
ORIGINAL	CURRENT	CHANGE	AMOUNT REMAINING

FOOD LOG

DATE _____

WEIGHT _____

TIME	AMOUNT	FOOD	CALORIES	PROTEIN	FAT	CARBS	FIBER	SODIUM
		TOTALS						
		GOALS						

VITAMINS/SUPPLEMENTS

_____

_____

8-ounce glasses of water

EXERCISE LOG

CARDIO				
ACTIVITY	LEVEL	DISTANCE	MINUTES	CALS BURNED

WEIGHTS			
ACTIVITY	WEIGHT	REPS	CALS BURNED

GOAL TRACKER			
ORIGINAL	CURRENT	CHANGE	AMOUNT REMAINING

FOOD LOG

DATE _____

WEIGHT _____

TIME	AMOUNT	FOOD	CALORIES	PROTEIN	FAT	CARBS	FIBER	SODIUM	
		TOTALS							
		GOALS							

VITAMINS/SUPPLEMENTS

_____

_____

8-ounce glasses of water

EXERCISE LOG

CARDIO				
ACTIVITY	LEVEL	DISTANCE	MINUTES	CALS BURNED

WEIGHTS			
ACTIVITY	WEIGHT	REPS	CALS BURNED

GOAL TRACKER			
ORIGINAL	CURRENT	CHANGE	AMOUNT REMAINING

FOOD LOG

DATE _____

WEIGHT _____

TIME	AMOUNT	FOOD	CALORIES	PROTEIN	FAT	CARBS	FIBER	SODIUM
		TOTALS						
		GOALS						

VITAMINS/SUPPLEMENTS

_____

_____

8-ounce glasses of water

EXERCISE LOG

CARDIO				
ACTIVITY	LEVEL	DISTANCE	MINUTES	CALS BURNED

WEIGHTS			
ACTIVITY	WEIGHT	REPS	CALS BURNED

GOAL TRACKER			
ORIGINAL	CURRENT	CHANGE	AMOUNT REMAINING

FOOD LOG

DATE _____

WEIGHT _____

TIME	AMOUNT	FOOD	CALORIES	PROTEIN	FAT	CARBS	FIBER	SODIUM	
		TOTALS							
		GOALS							

VITAMINS/SUPPLEMENTS

_____

_____

8-ounce glasses of water

EXERCISE LOG

CARDIO

ACTIVITY	LEVEL	DISTANCE	MINUTES	CALS BURNED

WEIGHTS

ACTIVITY	WEIGHT	REPS	CALS BURNED

GOAL TRACKER

ORIGINAL	CURRENT	CHANGE	AMOUNT REMAINING

FOOD LOG

DATE _____

WEIGHT _____

TIME	AMOUNT	FOOD	CALORIES	PROTEIN	FAT	CARBS	FIBER	SODIUM
		TOTALS						
		GOALS						

VITAMINS/SUPPLEMENTS

_____

_____

8-ounce glasses of water

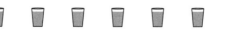

EXERCISE LOG

CARDIO				
ACTIVITY	LEVEL	DISTANCE	MINUTES	CALS BURNED

WEIGHTS			
ACTIVITY	WEIGHT	REPS	CALS BURNED

GOAL TRACKER			
ORIGINAL	CURRENT	CHANGE	AMOUNT REMAINING

FOOD LOG

DATE _____

WEIGHT _____

TIME	AMOUNT	FOOD	CALORIES	PROTEIN	FAT	CARBS	FIBER	SODIUM
		TOTALS						
		GOALS						

VITAMINS/SUPPLEMENTS

_____

_____

8-ounce glasses of water

EXERCISE LOG

CARDIO				
ACTIVITY	LEVEL	DISTANCE	MINUTES	CALS BURNED

WEIGHTS			
ACTIVITY	WEIGHT	REPS	CALS BURNED

GOAL TRACKER			
ORIGINAL	CURRENT	CHANGE	AMOUNT REMAINING

FOOD LOG

DATE _____

WEIGHT _____

TIME	AMOUNT	FOOD	CALORIES	PROTEIN	FAT	CARBS	FIBER	SODIUM
		TOTALS						
		GOALS						

VITAMINS/SUPPLEMENTS

8-ounce glasses of water

EXERCISE LOG

CARDIO

ACTIVITY	LEVEL	DISTANCE	MINUTES	CALS BURNED

WEIGHTS

ACTIVITY	WEIGHT	REPS	CALS BURNED

GOAL TRACKER

ORIGINAL	CURRENT	CHANGE	AMOUNT REMAINING

FOOD LOG

DATE _____

WEIGHT _____

TIME	AMOUNT	FOOD	CALORIES	PROTEIN	FAT	CARBS	FIBER	SODIUM
		TOTALS						
		GOALS						

VITAMINS/SUPPLEMENTS

_____

_____

8-ounce glasses of water

EXERCISE LOG

CARDIO				
ACTIVITY	LEVEL	DISTANCE	MINUTES	CALS BURNED

WEIGHTS			
ACTIVITY	WEIGHT	REPS	CALS BURNED

GOAL TRACKER			
ORIGINAL	CURRENT	CHANGE	AMOUNT REMAINING

FOOD LOG

DATE _____

WEIGHT _____

TIME	AMOUNT	FOOD	CALORIES	PROTEIN	FAT	CARBS	FIBER	SODIUM
		TOTALS						
		GOALS						

VITAMINS/SUPPLEMENTS

_____

_____

8-ounce glasses of water

EXERCISE LOG

CARDIO				
ACTIVITY	LEVEL	DISTANCE	MINUTES	CALS BURNED

WEIGHTS			
ACTIVITY	WEIGHT	REPS	CALS BURNED

GOAL TRACKER			
ORIGINAL	CURRENT	CHANGE	AMOUNT REMAINING

FOOD LOG

DATE _____

WEIGHT _____

TIME	AMOUNT	FOOD	CALORIES	PROTEIN	FAT	CARBS	FIBER	SODIUM
		TOTALS						
		GOALS						

VITAMINS/SUPPLEMENTS

_____

_____

8-ounce glasses of water

EXERCISE LOG

CARDIO				
ACTIVITY	LEVEL	DISTANCE	MINUTES	CALS BURNED

WEIGHTS			
ACTIVITY	WEIGHT	REPS	CALS BURNED

GOAL TRACKER			
ORIGINAL	CURRENT	CHANGE	AMOUNT REMAINING

FOOD LOG

DATE _____

WEIGHT _____

TIME	AMOUNT	FOOD	CALORIES	PROTEIN	FAT	CARBS	FIBER	SODIUM	
		TOTALS							
		GOALS							

VITAMINS/SUPPLEMENTS

_____

_____

8-ounce glasses of water

EXERCISE LOG

CARDIO				
ACTIVITY	LEVEL	DISTANCE	MINUTES	CALS BURNED

WEIGHTS			
ACTIVITY	WEIGHT	REPS	CALS BURNED

GOAL TRACKER			
ORIGINAL	CURRENT	CHANGE	AMOUNT REMAINING

FOOD LOG

DATE _____

WEIGHT _____

TIME	AMOUNT	FOOD	CALORIES	PROTEIN	FAT	CARBS	FIBER	SODIUM
		TOTALS						
		GOALS						

VITAMINS/SUPPLEMENTS

_____

_____

8-ounce glasses of water

EXERCISE LOG

CARDIO				
ACTIVITY	LEVEL	DISTANCE	MINUTES	CALS BURNED

WEIGHTS			
ACTIVITY	WEIGHT	REPS	CALS BURNED

GOAL TRACKER			
ORIGINAL	CURRENT	CHANGE	AMOUNT REMAINING

FOOD LOG

DATE _____

WEIGHT _____

TIME	AMOUNT	FOOD	CALORIES	PROTEIN	FAT	CARBS	FIBER	SODIUM
		TOTALS						
		GOALS						

VITAMINS/SUPPLEMENTS

_____

_____

8-ounce glasses of water

EXERCISE LOG

CARDIO				
ACTIVITY	LEVEL	DISTANCE	MINUTES	CALS BURNED

WEIGHTS			
ACTIVITY	WEIGHT	REPS	CALS BURNED

GOAL TRACKER			
ORIGINAL	CURRENT	CHANGE	AMOUNT REMAINING

FOOD LOG

DATE _____

WEIGHT _____

TIME	AMOUNT	FOOD	CALORIES	PROTEIN	FAT	CARBS	FIBER	SODIUM	
		TOTALS							
		GOALS							

VITAMINS/SUPPLEMENTS

_____

_____

8-ounce glasses of water

EXERCISE LOG

CARDIO				
ACTIVITY	LEVEL	DISTANCE	MINUTES	CALS BURNED

WEIGHTS			
ACTIVITY	WEIGHT	REPS	CALS BURNED

GOAL TRACKER			
ORIGINAL	CURRENT	CHANGE	AMOUNT REMAINING

FOOD LOG

DATE _____

WEIGHT _____

TIME	AMOUNT	FOOD	CALORIES	PROTEIN	FAT	CARBS	FIBER	SODIUM	
		TOTALS							
		GOALS							

VITAMINS/SUPPLEMENTS

8-ounce glasses of water

EXERCISE LOG

CARDIO				
ACTIVITY	LEVEL	DISTANCE	MINUTES	CALS BURNED

WEIGHTS			
ACTIVITY	WEIGHT	REPS	CALS BURNED

GOAL TRACKER			
ORIGINAL	CURRENT	CHANGE	AMOUNT REMAINING

FOOD LOG

DATE _____

WEIGHT _____

TIME	AMOUNT	FOOD	CALORIES	PROTEIN	FAT	CARBS	FIBER	SODIUM	
		TOTALS							
		GOALS							

VITAMINS/SUPPLEMENTS

_____

_____

8-ounce glasses of water

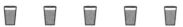

EXERCISE LOG

CARDIO				
ACTIVITY	LEVEL	DISTANCE	MINUTES	CALS BURNED

WEIGHTS			
ACTIVITY	WEIGHT	REPS	CALS BURNED

GOAL TRACKER			
ORIGINAL	CURRENT	CHANGE	AMOUNT REMAINING

FOOD LOG

DATE _____

WEIGHT _____

TIME	AMOUNT	FOOD	CALORIES	PROTEIN	FAT	CARBS	FIBER	SODIUM
		TOTALS						
		GOALS						

VITAMINS/SUPPLEMENTS

_____

_____

8-ounce glasses of water

EXERCISE LOG

CARDIO

ACTIVITY	LEVEL	DISTANCE	MINUTES	CALS BURNED

WEIGHTS

ACTIVITY	WEIGHT	REPS	CALS BURNED

GOAL TRACKER

ORIGINAL	CURRENT	CHANGE	AMOUNT REMAINING

FOOD LOG

DATE _____

WEIGHT _____

TIME	AMOUNT	FOOD	CALORIES	PROTEIN	FAT	CARBS	FIBER	SODIUM
		TOTALS						
		GOALS						

VITAMINS/SUPPLEMENTS

_____

_____

8-ounce glasses of water

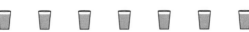

88

EXERCISE LOG

CARDIO				
ACTIVITY	LEVEL	DISTANCE	MINUTES	CALS BURNED

WEIGHTS			
ACTIVITY	WEIGHT	REPS	CALS BURNED

GOAL TRACKER			
ORIGINAL	CURRENT	CHANGE	AMOUNT REMAINING

FOOD LOG

DATE _____

WEIGHT _____

TIME	AMOUNT	FOOD	CALORIES	PROTEIN	FAT	CARBS	FIBER	SODIUM	
		TOTALS							
		GOALS							

VITAMINS/SUPPLEMENTS

_____

_____

8-ounce glasses of water

EXERCISE LOG

CARDIO				
ACTIVITY	LEVEL	DISTANCE	MINUTES	CALS BURNED

WEIGHTS			
ACTIVITY	WEIGHT	REPS	CALS BURNED

GOAL TRACKER			
ORIGINAL	CURRENT	CHANGE	AMOUNT REMAINING

FOOD LOG

DATE _____

WEIGHT _____

TIME	AMOUNT	FOOD	CALORIES	PROTEIN	FAT	CARBS	FIBER	SODIUM	
		TOTALS							
		GOALS							

VITAMINS/SUPPLEMENTS

8-ounce glasses of water

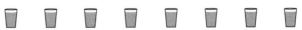

EXERCISE LOG

CARDIO

ACTIVITY	LEVEL	DISTANCE	MINUTES	CALS BURNED

WEIGHTS

ACTIVITY	WEIGHT	REPS	CALS BURNED

GOAL TRACKER

ORIGINAL	CURRENT	CHANGE	AMOUNT REMAINING

FOOD LOG

DATE _____

WEIGHT _____

TIME	AMOUNT	FOOD	CALORIES	PROTEIN	FAT	CARBS	FIBER	SODIUM
		TOTALS						
		GOALS						

VITAMINS/SUPPLEMENTS

_____

_____

8-ounce glasses of water

EXERCISE LOG

CARDIO

ACTIVITY	LEVEL	DISTANCE	MINUTES	CALS BURNED

WEIGHTS

ACTIVITY	WEIGHT	REPS	CALS BURNED

GOAL TRACKER

ORIGINAL	CURRENT	CHANGE	AMOUNT REMAINING

FOOD LOG

DATE _____

WEIGHT _____

TIME	AMOUNT	FOOD	CALORIES	PROTEIN	FAT	CARBS	FIBER	SODIUM
		TOTALS						
		GOALS						

VITAMINS/SUPPLEMENTS

_____

_____

8-ounce glasses of water

EXERCISE LOG

CARDIO				
ACTIVITY	LEVEL	DISTANCE	MINUTES	CALS BURNED

WEIGHTS			
ACTIVITY	WEIGHT	REPS	CALS BURNED

GOAL TRACKER			
ORIGINAL	CURRENT	CHANGE	AMOUNT REMAINING

FOOD LOG

DATE _____

WEIGHT _____

TIME	AMOUNT	FOOD	CALORIES	PROTEIN	FAT	CARBS	FIBER	SODIUM
		TOTALS						
		GOALS						

VITAMINS/SUPPLEMENTS

8-ounce glasses of water

EXERCISE LOG

CARDIO				
ACTIVITY	LEVEL	DISTANCE	MINUTES	CALS BURNED

WEIGHTS			
ACTIVITY	WEIGHT	REPS	CALS BURNED

GOAL TRACKER			
ORIGINAL	CURRENT	CHANGE	AMOUNT REMAINING

FOOD LOG

DATE _____

WEIGHT _____

TIME	AMOUNT	FOOD	CALORIES	PROTEIN	FAT	CARBS	FIBER	SODIUM	
		TOTALS							
		GOALS							

VITAMINS/SUPPLEMENTS

_____

_____

8-ounce glasses of water

EXERCISE LOG

CARDIO				
ACTIVITY	LEVEL	DISTANCE	MINUTES	CALS BURNED

WEIGHTS			
ACTIVITY	WEIGHT	REPS	CALS BURNED

GOAL TRACKER			
ORIGINAL	CURRENT	CHANGE	AMOUNT REMAINING

FOOD LOG

DATE _____

WEIGHT _____

TIME	AMOUNT	FOOD	CALORIES	PROTEIN	FAT	CARBS	FIBER	SODIUM
		TOTALS						
		GOALS						

VITAMINS/SUPPLEMENTS

_____

_____

8-ounce glasses of water

EXERCISE LOG

CARDIO				
ACTIVITY	LEVEL	DISTANCE	MINUTES	CALS BURNED

WEIGHTS			
ACTIVITY	WEIGHT	REPS	CALS BURNED

GOAL TRACKER			
ORIGINAL	CURRENT	CHANGE	AMOUNT REMAINING

FOOD LOG

DATE _____

WEIGHT _____

TIME	AMOUNT	FOOD	CALORIES	PROTEIN	FAT	CARBS	FIBER	SODIUM	
		TOTALS							
		GOALS							

VITAMINS/SUPPLEMENTS

8-ounce glasses of water

EXERCISE LOG

CARDIO

ACTIVITY	LEVEL	DISTANCE	MINUTES	CALS BURNED

WEIGHTS

ACTIVITY	WEIGHT	REPS	CALS BURNED

GOAL TRACKER

ORIGINAL	CURRENT	CHANGE	AMOUNT REMAINING

FOOD LOG

DATE _____

WEIGHT _____

TIME	AMOUNT	FOOD	CALORIES	PROTEIN	FAT	CARBS	FIBER	SODIUM	
		TOTALS							
		GOALS							

VITAMINS/SUPPLEMENTS

_____

_____

8-ounce glasses of water

EXERCISE LOG

CARDIO				
ACTIVITY	LEVEL	DISTANCE	MINUTES	CALS BURNED

WEIGHTS			
ACTIVITY	WEIGHT	REPS	CALS BURNED

GOAL TRACKER			
ORIGINAL	CURRENT	CHANGE	AMOUNT REMAINING

FOOD LOG

DATE _____

WEIGHT _____

TIME	AMOUNT	FOOD	CALORIES	PROTEIN	FAT	CARBS	FIBER	SODIUM
		TOTALS						
		GOALS						

VITAMINS/SUPPLEMENTS

_____

_____

8-ounce glasses of water

EXERCISE LOG

CARDIO				
ACTIVITY	LEVEL	DISTANCE	MINUTES	CALS BURNED

WEIGHTS			
ACTIVITY	WEIGHT	REPS	CALS BURNED

GOAL TRACKER			
ORIGINAL	CURRENT	CHANGE	AMOUNT REMAINING

FOOD LOG

DATE _____

WEIGHT _____

TIME	AMOUNT	FOOD	CALORIES	PROTEIN	FAT	CARBS	FIBER	SODIUM
		TOTALS						
		GOALS						

VITAMINS/SUPPLEMENTS

_____

_____

8-ounce glasses of water

EXERCISE LOG

CARDIO				
ACTIVITY	LEVEL	DISTANCE	MINUTES	CALS BURNED

WEIGHTS			
ACTIVITY	WEIGHT	REPS	CALS BURNED

GOAL TRACKER			
ORIGINAL	CURRENT	CHANGE	AMOUNT REMAINING

FOOD LOG

DATE _____

WEIGHT _____

TIME	AMOUNT	FOOD	CALORIES	PROTEIN	FAT	CARBS	FIBER	SODIUM	
		TOTALS							
		GOALS							

VITAMINS/SUPPLEMENTS

8-ounce glasses of water

EXERCISE LOG

CARDIO

ACTIVITY	LEVEL	DISTANCE	MINUTES	CALS BURNED

WEIGHTS

ACTIVITY	WEIGHT	REPS	CALS BURNED

GOAL TRACKER

ORIGINAL	CURRENT	CHANGE	AMOUNT REMAINING

FOOD LOG

DATE _____

WEIGHT _____

TIME	AMOUNT	FOOD	CALORIES	PROTEIN	FAT	CARBS	FIBER	SODIUM	
		TOTALS							
		GOALS							

VITAMINS/SUPPLEMENTS

_____

_____

8-ounce glasses of water

EXERCISE LOG

CARDIO

ACTIVITY	LEVEL	DISTANCE	MINUTES	CALS BURNED

WEIGHTS

ACTIVITY	WEIGHT	REPS	CALS BURNED

GOAL TRACKER

ORIGINAL	CURRENT	CHANGE	AMOUNT REMAINING

FOOD LOG

DATE _____

WEIGHT _____

TIME	AMOUNT	FOOD	CALORIES	PROTEIN	FAT	CARBS	FIBER	SODIUM	
		TOTALS							
		GOALS							

VITAMINS/SUPPLEMENTS

_____

_____

8-ounce glasses of water

EXERCISE LOG

CARDIO				
ACTIVITY	LEVEL	DISTANCE	MINUTES	CALS BURNED

WEIGHTS			
ACTIVITY	WEIGHT	REPS	CALS BURNED

GOAL TRACKER			
ORIGINAL	CURRENT	CHANGE	AMOUNT REMAINING

FOOD LOG

DATE _____

WEIGHT _____

TIME	AMOUNT	FOOD	CALORIES	PROTEIN	FAT	CARBS	FIBER	SODIUM
		TOTALS						
		GOALS						

VITAMINS/SUPPLEMENTS

8-ounce glasses of water

EXERCISE LOG

CARDIO				
ACTIVITY	LEVEL	DISTANCE	MINUTES	CALS BURNED

WEIGHTS			
ACTIVITY	WEIGHT	REPS	CALS BURNED

GOAL TRACKER			
ORIGINAL	CURRENT	CHANGE	AMOUNT REMAINING

FOOD LOG

DATE _____

WEIGHT _____

TIME	AMOUNT	FOOD	CALORIES	PROTEIN	FAT	CARBS	FIBER	SODIUM
		TOTALS						
		GOALS						

VITAMINS/SUPPLEMENTS

_____

_____

8-ounce glasses of water

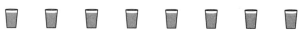

120

EXERCISE LOG

CARDIO				
ACTIVITY	LEVEL	DISTANCE	MINUTES	CALS BURNED

WEIGHTS			
ACTIVITY	WEIGHT	REPS	CALS BURNED

GOAL TRACKER			
ORIGINAL	CURRENT	CHANGE	AMOUNT REMAINING

FOOD LOG

DATE _____

WEIGHT _____

TIME	AMOUNT	FOOD	CALORIES	PROTEIN	FAT	CARBS	FIBER	SODIUM	
		TOTALS							
		GOALS							

VITAMINS/SUPPLEMENTS

8-ounce glasses of water

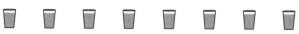

122

EXERCISE LOG

CARDIO				
ACTIVITY	LEVEL	DISTANCE	MINUTES	CALS BURNED

WEIGHTS			
ACTIVITY	WEIGHT	REPS	CALS BURNED

GOAL TRACKER			
ORIGINAL	CURRENT	CHANGE	AMOUNT REMAINING

FOOD LOG

DATE _____

WEIGHT _____

TIME	AMOUNT	FOOD	CALORIES	PROTEIN	FAT	CARBS	FIBER	SODIUM	
		TOTALS							
		GOALS							

VITAMINS/SUPPLEMENTS

_____

_____

8-ounce glasses of water

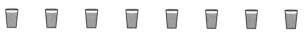

EXERCISE LOG

CARDIO				
ACTIVITY	LEVEL	DISTANCE	MINUTES	CALS BURNED

WEIGHTS			
ACTIVITY	WEIGHT	REPS	CALS BURNED

GOAL TRACKER			
ORIGINAL	CURRENT	CHANGE	AMOUNT REMAINING

FOOD LOG

DATE _____

WEIGHT _____

TIME	AMOUNT	FOOD	CALORIES	PROTEIN	FAT	CARBS	FIBER	SODIUM
		TOTALS						
		GOALS						

VITAMINS/SUPPLEMENTS

_____

_____

8-ounce glasses of water

EXERCISE LOG

CARDIO

ACTIVITY	LEVEL	DISTANCE	MINUTES	CALS BURNED

WEIGHTS

ACTIVITY	WEIGHT	REPS	CALS BURNED

GOAL TRACKER

ORIGINAL	CURRENT	CHANGE	AMOUNT REMAINING

FOOD LOG

DATE _____

WEIGHT _____

TIME	AMOUNT	FOOD	CALORIES	PROTEIN	FAT	CARBS	FIBER	SODIUM	
		TOTALS							
		GOALS							

VITAMINS/SUPPLEMENTS

_____

_____

8-ounce glasses of water

EXERCISE LOG

CARDIO

ACTIVITY	LEVEL	DISTANCE	MINUTES	CALS BURNED

WEIGHTS

ACTIVITY	WEIGHT	REPS	CALS BURNED

GOAL TRACKER

ORIGINAL	CURRENT	CHANGE	AMOUNT REMAINING

FOOD LOG

DATE _____

WEIGHT _____

TIME	AMOUNT	FOOD	CALORIES	PROTEIN	FAT	CARBS	FIBER	SODIUM
		TOTALS						
		GOALS						

VITAMINS/SUPPLEMENTS

8-ounce glasses of water

EXERCISE LOG

CARDIO				
ACTIVITY	LEVEL	DISTANCE	MINUTES	CALS BURNED

WEIGHTS			
ACTIVITY	WEIGHT	REPS	CALS BURNED

GOAL TRACKER			
ORIGINAL	CURRENT	CHANGE	AMOUNT REMAINING

FOOD LOG

DATE _____

WEIGHT _____

TIME	AMOUNT	FOOD	CALORIES	PROTEIN	FAT	CARBS	FIBER	SODIUM	
		TOTALS							
		GOALS							

VITAMINS/SUPPLEMENTS

_____

_____

8-ounce glasses of water

EXERCISE LOG

CARDIO				
ACTIVITY	LEVEL	DISTANCE	MINUTES	CALS BURNED

WEIGHTS			
ACTIVITY	WEIGHT	REPS	CALS BURNED

GOAL TRACKER			
ORIGINAL	CURRENT	CHANGE	AMOUNT REMAINING

FOOD LOG

DATE _____

WEIGHT _____

TIME	AMOUNT	FOOD	CALORIES	PROTEIN	FAT	CARBS	FIBER	SODIUM	
		TOTALS							
		GOALS							

VITAMINS/SUPPLEMENTS

8-ounce glasses of water

EXERCISE LOG

CARDIO				
ACTIVITY	LEVEL	DISTANCE	MINUTES	CALS BURNED

WEIGHTS			
ACTIVITY	WEIGHT	REPS	CALS BURNED

GOAL TRACKER			
ORIGINAL	CURRENT	CHANGE	AMOUNT REMAINING

FOOD LOG

DATE _____

WEIGHT _____

TIME	AMOUNT	FOOD	CALORIES	PROTEIN	FAT	CARBS	FIBER	SODIUM
		TOTALS						
		GOALS						

VITAMINS/SUPPLEMENTS

_____

_____

8-ounce glasses of water

EXERCISE LOG

CARDIO				
ACTIVITY	LEVEL	DISTANCE	MINUTES	CALS BURNED

WEIGHTS			
ACTIVITY	WEIGHT	REPS	CALS BURNED

GOAL TRACKER			
ORIGINAL	CURRENT	CHANGE	AMOUNT REMAINING

FOOD LOG

DATE _____

WEIGHT _____

TIME	AMOUNT	FOOD	CALORIES	PROTEIN	FAT	CARBS	FIBER	SODIUM
		TOTALS						
		GOALS						

VITAMINS/SUPPLEMENTS

8-ounce glasses of water

EXERCISE LOG

CARDIO				
ACTIVITY	LEVEL	DISTANCE	MINUTES	CALS BURNED

WEIGHTS			
ACTIVITY	WEIGHT	REPS	CALS BURNED

GOAL TRACKER			
ORIGINAL	CURRENT	CHANGE	AMOUNT REMAINING

FOOD LOG

DATE _____

WEIGHT _____

TIME	AMOUNT	FOOD	CALORIES	PROTEIN	FAT	CARBS	FIBER	SODIUM	
		TOTALS							
		GOALS							

VITAMINS/SUPPLEMENTS

_____

_____

8-ounce glasses of water

EXERCISE LOG

CARDIO				
ACTIVITY	LEVEL	DISTANCE	MINUTES	CALS BURNED

WEIGHTS			
ACTIVITY	WEIGHT	REPS	CALS BURNED

GOAL TRACKER			
ORIGINAL	CURRENT	CHANGE	AMOUNT REMAINING

FOOD LOG

DATE _____

WEIGHT _____

TIME	AMOUNT	FOOD	CALORIES	PROTEIN	FAT	CARBS	FIBER	SODIUM
		TOTALS						
		GOALS						

VITAMINS/SUPPLEMENTS

8-ounce glasses of water

EXERCISE LOG

CARDIO				
ACTIVITY	LEVEL	DISTANCE	MINUTES	CALS BURNED

WEIGHTS			
ACTIVITY	WEIGHT	REPS	CALS BURNED

GOAL TRACKER			
ORIGINAL	CURRENT	CHANGE	AMOUNT REMAINING

FOOD LOG

DATE _____

WEIGHT _____

TIME	AMOUNT	FOOD	CALORIES	PROTEIN	FAT	CARBS	FIBER	SODIUM
		TOTALS						
		GOALS						

VITAMINS/SUPPLEMENTS

_____

_____

8-ounce glasses of water

EXERCISE LOG

CARDIO				
ACTIVITY	LEVEL	DISTANCE	MINUTES	CALS BURNED

WEIGHTS			
ACTIVITY	WEIGHT	REPS	CALS BURNED

GOAL TRACKER			
ORIGINAL	CURRENT	CHANGE	AMOUNT REMAINING

FOOD LOG

DATE _____

WEIGHT _____

TIME	AMOUNT	FOOD	CALORIES	PROTEIN	FAT	CARBS	FIBER	SODIUM	
		TOTALS							
		GOALS							

VITAMINS/SUPPLEMENTS

8-ounce glasses of water

EXERCISE LOG

CARDIO				
ACTIVITY	LEVEL	DISTANCE	MINUTES	CALS BURNED

WEIGHTS			
ACTIVITY	WEIGHT	REPS	CALS BURNED

GOAL TRACKER			
ORIGINAL	CURRENT	CHANGE	AMOUNT REMAINING

FOOD LOG

DATE _____

WEIGHT _____

TIME	AMOUNT	FOOD	CALORIES	PROTEIN	FAT	CARBS	FIBER	SODIUM
		TOTALS						
		GOALS						

VITAMINS/SUPPLEMENTS

_____

_____

8-ounce glasses of water

EXERCISE LOG

CARDIO

ACTIVITY	LEVEL	DISTANCE	MINUTES	CALS BURNED

WEIGHTS

ACTIVITY	WEIGHT	REPS	CALS BURNED

GOAL TRACKER

ORIGINAL	CURRENT	CHANGE	AMOUNT REMAINING

FOOD LOG

DATE _____

WEIGHT _____

TIME	AMOUNT	FOOD	CALORIES	PROTEIN	FAT	CARBS	FIBER	SODIUM	
		TOTALS							
		GOALS							

VITAMINS/SUPPLEMENTS

_____

_____

8-ounce glasses of water

EXERCISE LOG

CARDIO				
ACTIVITY	LEVEL	DISTANCE	MINUTES	CALS BURNED

WEIGHTS			
ACTIVITY	WEIGHT	REPS	CALS BURNED

GOAL TRACKER			
ORIGINAL	CURRENT	CHANGE	AMOUNT REMAINING

FOOD LOG

DATE _____

WEIGHT _____

TIME	AMOUNT	FOOD	CALORIES	PROTEIN	FAT	CARBS	FIBER	SODIUM	
		TOTALS							
		GOALS							

VITAMINS/SUPPLEMENTS

_____

_____

8-ounce glasses of water

EXERCISE LOG

CARDIO

ACTIVITY	LEVEL	DISTANCE	MINUTES	CALS BURNED

WEIGHTS

ACTIVITY	WEIGHT	REPS	CALS BURNED

GOAL TRACKER

ORIGINAL	CURRENT	CHANGE	AMOUNT REMAINING

FOOD LOG

DATE _____

WEIGHT _____

TIME	AMOUNT	FOOD	CALORIES	PROTEIN	FAT	CARBS	FIBER	SODIUM
		TOTALS						
		GOALS						

VITAMINS/SUPPLEMENTS

_____

_____

8-ounce glasses of water

EXERCISE LOG

CARDIO				
ACTIVITY	LEVEL	DISTANCE	MINUTES	CALS BURNED

WEIGHTS			
ACTIVITY	WEIGHT	REPS	CALS BURNED

GOAL TRACKER			
ORIGINAL	CURRENT	CHANGE	AMOUNT REMAINING

FOOD LOG

DATE _____

WEIGHT _____

TIME	AMOUNT	FOOD	CALORIES	PROTEIN	FAT	CARBS	FIBER	SODIUM
		TOTALS						
		GOALS						

VITAMINS/SUPPLEMENTS

_____

_____

8-ounce glasses of water

EXERCISE LOG

CARDIO				
ACTIVITY	LEVEL	DISTANCE	MINUTES	CALS BURNED

WEIGHTS			
ACTIVITY	WEIGHT	REPS	CALS BURNED

GOAL TRACKER			
ORIGINAL	CURRENT	CHANGE	AMOUNT REMAINING

FOOD LOG

DATE _____

WEIGHT _____

TIME	AMOUNT	FOOD	CALORIES	PROTEIN	FAT	CARBS	FIBER	SODIUM
		TOTALS						
		GOALS						

VITAMINS/SUPPLEMENTS

_____

_____

8-ounce glasses of water

EXERCISE LOG

CARDIO				
ACTIVITY	LEVEL	DISTANCE	MINUTES	CALS BURNED

WEIGHTS			
ACTIVITY	WEIGHT	REPS	CALS BURNED

GOAL TRACKER			
ORIGINAL	CURRENT	CHANGE	AMOUNT REMAINING

FOOD LOG

DATE _____

WEIGHT _____

TIME	AMOUNT	FOOD	CALORIES	PROTEIN	FAT	CARBS	FIBER	SODIUM
		TOTALS						
		GOALS						

VITAMINS/SUPPLEMENTS

_____

_____

8-ounce glasses of water

EXERCISE LOG

CARDIO

ACTIVITY	LEVEL	DISTANCE	MINUTES	CALS BURNED

WEIGHTS

ACTIVITY	WEIGHT	REPS	CALS BURNED

GOAL TRACKER

ORIGINAL	CURRENT	CHANGE	AMOUNT REMAINING

FOOD LOG

DATE _____

WEIGHT _____

TIME	AMOUNT	FOOD	CALORIES	PROTEIN	FAT	CARBS	FIBER	SODIUM	
		TOTALS							
		GOALS							

VITAMINS/SUPPLEMENTS

_____

_____

8-ounce glasses of water

EXERCISE LOG

CARDIO				
ACTIVITY	LEVEL	DISTANCE	MINUTES	CALS BURNED

WEIGHTS			
ACTIVITY	WEIGHT	REPS	CALS BURNED

GOAL TRACKER			
ORIGINAL	CURRENT	CHANGE	AMOUNT REMAINING

FOOD LOG

DATE _____

WEIGHT _____

TIME	AMOUNT	FOOD	CALORIES	PROTEIN	FAT	CARBS	FIBER	SODIUM
		TOTALS						
		GOALS						

VITAMINS/SUPPLEMENTS

_____

_____

8-ounce glasses of water

EXERCISE LOG

CARDIO

ACTIVITY	LEVEL	DISTANCE	MINUTES	CALS BURNED

WEIGHTS

ACTIVITY	WEIGHT	REPS	CALS BURNED

GOAL TRACKER

ORIGINAL	CURRENT	CHANGE	AMOUNT REMAINING

FOOD LOG

DATE _____

WEIGHT _____

TIME	AMOUNT	FOOD	CALORIES	PROTEIN	FAT	CARBS	FIBER	SODIUM
		TOTALS						
		GOALS						

VITAMINS/SUPPLEMENTS

_____

_____

8-ounce glasses of water

EXERCISE LOG

CARDIO				
ACTIVITY	LEVEL	DISTANCE	MINUTES	CALS BURNED

WEIGHTS			
ACTIVITY	WEIGHT	REPS	CALS BURNED

GOAL TRACKER			
ORIGINAL	CURRENT	CHANGE	AMOUNT REMAINING

FOOD LOG

DATE _____

WEIGHT _____

TIME	AMOUNT	FOOD	CALORIES	PROTEIN	FAT	CARBS	FIBER	SODIUM	
		TOTALS							
		GOALS							

VITAMINS/SUPPLEMENTS

_____

_____

8-ounce glasses of water

EXERCISE LOG

CARDIO				
ACTIVITY	LEVEL	DISTANCE	MINUTES	CALS BURNED

WEIGHTS			
ACTIVITY	WEIGHT	REPS	CALS BURNED

GOAL TRACKER			
ORIGINAL	CURRENT	CHANGE	AMOUNT REMAINING

FOOD LOG

DATE _____

WEIGHT _____

TIME	AMOUNT	FOOD	CALORIES	PROTEIN	FAT	CARBS	FIBER	SODIUM
		TOTALS						
		GOALS						

VITAMINS/SUPPLEMENTS

_____

_____

8-ounce glasses of water

EXERCISE LOG

CARDIO				
ACTIVITY	LEVEL	DISTANCE	MINUTES	CALS BURNED

WEIGHTS			
ACTIVITY	WEIGHT	REPS	CALS BURNED

GOAL TRACKER			
ORIGINAL	CURRENT	CHANGE	AMOUNT REMAINING

FOOD LOG

DATE _____

WEIGHT _____

TIME	AMOUNT	FOOD	CALORIES	PROTEIN	FAT	CARBS	FIBER	SODIUM
		TOTALS						
		GOALS						

VITAMINS/SUPPLEMENTS

_____

_____

8-ounce glasses of water

EXERCISE LOG

CARDIO				
ACTIVITY	LEVEL	DISTANCE	MINUTES	CALS BURNED

WEIGHTS			
ACTIVITY	WEIGHT	REPS	CALS BURNED

GOAL TRACKER			
ORIGINAL	CURRENT	CHANGE	AMOUNT REMAINING

FOOD LOG

DATE _____

WEIGHT _____

TIME	AMOUNT	FOOD	CALORIES	PROTEIN	FAT	CARBS	FIBER	SODIUM
		TOTALS						
		GOALS						

VITAMINS/SUPPLEMENTS

_____

_____

8-ounce glasses of water

EXERCISE LOG

CARDIO				
ACTIVITY	LEVEL	DISTANCE	MINUTES	CALS BURNED

WEIGHTS			
ACTIVITY	WEIGHT	REPS	CALS BURNED

GOAL TRACKER			
ORIGINAL	CURRENT	CHANGE	AMOUNT REMAINING

FOOD LOG

DATE _____

WEIGHT _____

TIME	AMOUNT	FOOD	CALORIES	PROTEIN	FAT	CARBS	FIBER	SODIUM
		TOTALS						
		GOALS						

VITAMINS/SUPPLEMENTS

_____

_____

8-ounce glasses of water

EXERCISE LOG

CARDIO				
ACTIVITY	LEVEL	DISTANCE	MINUTES	CALS BURNED

WEIGHTS			
ACTIVITY	WEIGHT	REPS	CALS BURNED

GOAL TRACKER			
ORIGINAL	CURRENT	CHANGE	AMOUNT REMAINING

FOOD LOG

DATE _____

WEIGHT _____

TIME	AMOUNT	FOOD	CALORIES	PROTEIN	FAT	CARBS	FIBER	SODIUM	
		TOTALS							
		GOALS							

VITAMINS/SUPPLEMENTS

_____

_____

8-ounce glasses of water

EXERCISE LOG

CARDIO				
ACTIVITY	LEVEL	DISTANCE	MINUTES	CALS BURNED

WEIGHTS			
ACTIVITY	WEIGHT	REPS	CALS BURNED

GOAL TRACKER			
ORIGINAL	CURRENT	CHANGE	AMOUNT REMAINING

FOOD LOG

DATE _____

WEIGHT _____

TIME	AMOUNT	FOOD	CALORIES	PROTEIN	FAT	CARBS	FIBER	SODIUM
		TOTALS						
		GOALS						

VITAMINS/SUPPLEMENTS

_____

_____

8-ounce glasses of water

EXERCISE LOG

CARDIO				
ACTIVITY	LEVEL	DISTANCE	MINUTES	CALS BURNED

WEIGHTS			
ACTIVITY	WEIGHT	REPS	CALS BURNED

GOAL TRACKER			
ORIGINAL	CURRENT	CHANGE	AMOUNT REMAINING

FOOD LOG

DATE _____

WEIGHT _____

TIME	AMOUNT	FOOD	CALORIES	PROTEIN	FAT	CARBS	FIBER	SODIUM
		TOTALS						
		GOALS						

VITAMINS/SUPPLEMENTS

_____

_____

8-ounce glasses of water

EXERCISE LOG

CARDIO				
ACTIVITY	LEVEL	DISTANCE	MINUTES	CALS BURNED

WEIGHTS			
ACTIVITY	WEIGHT	REPS	CALS BURNED

GOAL TRACKER			
ORIGINAL	CURRENT	CHANGE	AMOUNT REMAINING

FOOD LOG

DATE _____

WEIGHT _____

TIME	AMOUNT	FOOD	CALORIES	PROTEIN	FAT	CARBS	FIBER	SODIUM
		TOTALS						
		GOALS						

VITAMINS/SUPPLEMENTS

_____

_____

8-ounce glasses of water

EXERCISE LOG

CARDIO				
ACTIVITY	LEVEL	DISTANCE	MINUTES	CALS BURNED

WEIGHTS			
ACTIVITY	WEIGHT	REPS	CALS BURNED

GOAL TRACKER			
ORIGINAL	CURRENT	CHANGE	AMOUNT REMAINING

FOOD LOG

DATE _____

WEIGHT _____

TIME	AMOUNT	FOOD	CALORIES	PROTEIN	FAT	CARBS	FIBER	SODIUM
		TOTALS						
		GOALS						

VITAMINS/SUPPLEMENTS

_____

_____

8-ounce glasses of water

EXERCISE LOG

CARDIO				
ACTIVITY	LEVEL	DISTANCE	MINUTES	CALS BURNED

WEIGHTS			
ACTIVITY	WEIGHT	REPS	CALS BURNED

GOAL TRACKER			
ORIGINAL	CURRENT	CHANGE	AMOUNT REMAINING

FOOD LOG

DATE _____

WEIGHT _____

TIME	AMOUNT	FOOD	CALORIES	PROTEIN	FAT	CARBS	FIBER	SODIUM
		TOTALS						
		GOALS						

VITAMINS/SUPPLEMENTS

_____

_____

8-ounce glasses of water

EXERCISE LOG

CARDIO				
ACTIVITY	LEVEL	DISTANCE	MINUTES	CALS BURNED

WEIGHTS			
ACTIVITY	WEIGHT	REPS	CALS BURNED

GOAL TRACKER			
ORIGINAL	CURRENT	CHANGE	AMOUNT REMAINING

FOOD LOG

DATE _____

WEIGHT _____

TIME	AMOUNT	FOOD	CALORIES	PROTEIN	FAT	CARBS	FIBER	SODIUM	
		TOTALS							
		GOALS							

VITAMINS/SUPPLEMENTS

8-ounce glasses of water

EXERCISE LOG

CARDIO				
ACTIVITY	LEVEL	DISTANCE	MINUTES	CALS BURNED

WEIGHTS			
ACTIVITY	WEIGHT	REPS	CALS BURNED

GOAL TRACKER			
ORIGINAL	CURRENT	CHANGE	AMOUNT REMAINING

PROGRESS CHARTS

As they say, a picture is worth a thousand words! The following graphs allow you to track your weekly progress visually. Take any statistics from your **WEEKLY STATISTICS** tables and plot them on the graphs on the following pages. You can even use the same graph to plot two different groups of data, as our sample dieter did in the graphs below, for easy comparison.

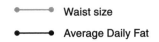

Waist size

Average Daily Fat

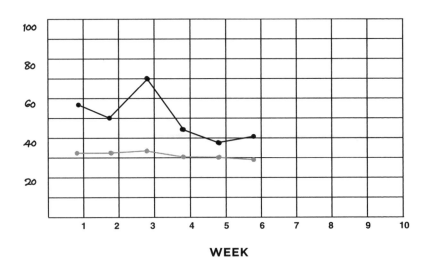

WEEK

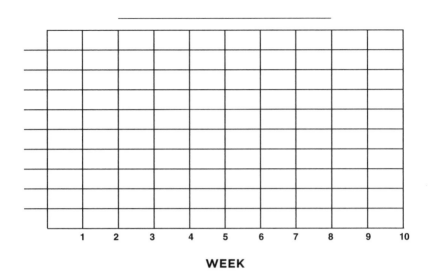

WEEK

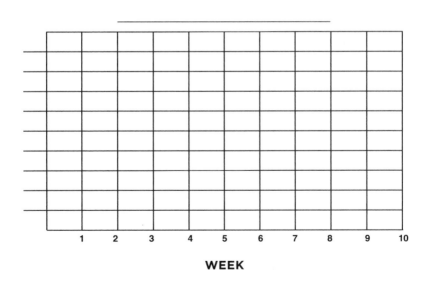

WEEK

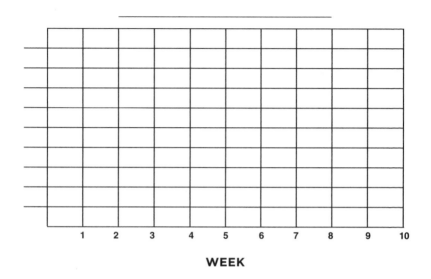

WEEK

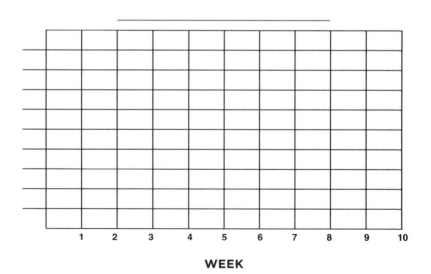

WEEK

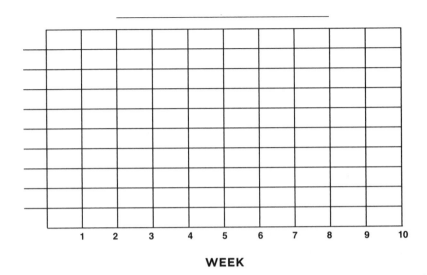

WEEK

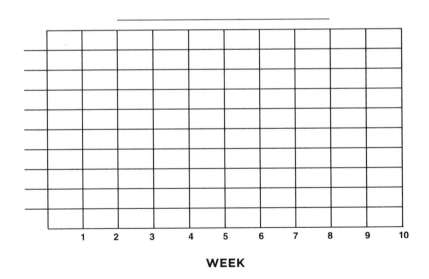

WEEK

NUTRIENT TABLE

Food	Serving	Cals	Protein (g)	Fat (g)	Carbs (g)	Fiber (g)	Sodium (mg)	Cholesterol (mg)	Calcium (mg)	Vit D (IU)	Iron (mg)	Potassium (mg)
acai berry drk, fort	8 fl oz	62	0.83	0.83	12.83	1.2	13	0	19	0	0.16	130
agave, ckd (southwest)	100 g	135	0.99	0.29	32	10.6	13	0	460	0	3.55	59
agave, dried (southwest)	100 g	341	1.71	0.69	81.98	15.6	14	0	770	0	3.64	767
agave, raw (southwest)	100 g	68	0.52	0.15	16.23	6.6	14	0	417	0	1.8	127
alcohol (gin, rum, vodka, whiskey) 80 proof	1 fl oz	231	0	0	0	0	1	0	0	0	0.04	2
alcohol (gin, rum, vodka, whiskey) 90 proof	1 fl oz	263	0	0	0	0	1	0	0	0	0.04	2
allspice, ground	1 tsp	263	6.09	8.69	72.12	21.6	77	0	661	0	7.06	1044
almond butter, pln, w/salt	1 tbsp	614	20.96	55.5	18.82	10.3	227	0	347	0	3.49	748
almond butter, pln, wo/salt	1 tbsp	614	20.96	55.5	18.82	10.3	7	0	347	0	3.49	748
almond milk, choc, rtd	8 fl oz	50	0.63	1.25	9.38	0.4	71	0	188	42	0.53	75
almond milk, swtnd, vanilla flavor, rtd	8 fl oz	38	0.42	1.04	6.59	0.4	63	0	188	42	0.3	50
almond milk, unswtnd, shelf stable	1 cup	15	0.59	1.1	0.58	0	71	0	197	42	0.35	67
almonds	1 cup	579	21.15	49.93	21.55	12.5	1	0	269	0	3.71	733
almonds, oil rstd, lightly salted	1 cup	607	21.23	55.17	17.68	10.5	143	0	291		3.68	699
almonds, oil rstd, w/ salt added, smoke flavor	1 oz	607	21.43	55.89	17.86	10.7	548	0	286		3.86	679
aloe vera juc drk, fort w/ vit c	8 fl oz	15	0	0	3.75	0	8	0	8	0	0.15	0
amber, hard cider	12 fl oz	56	0	0	5.92	0	4	0	4	0	0.06	54
animal fat, bacon grease	1 tsp	897	0	99.5	0	0	150	95	0	101	0	0
appl crisp, prepared-from-recipe	.5 cup	161	1.75	3.43	30.84	1.4	351	0	35		0.82	78
appl juc drk, lt, fort w/ vit c	8 fl oz	22	0	0.1	5.1	0	13	0	3	0	0.2	51
apple juc, cnd or bltd, unswtnd, w/ added vit c	1 cup	46	0.1	0.13	11.3	0.2	4	0	8	0	0.12	101
apples, raw, with skin	1 cup	52	0.26	0.17	13.81	2.4	1	0	6	0	0.12	107
apples, raw, without skin	1 cup, slices	48	0.27	0.13	12.76	1.3	0	0	5	0	0.07	90
applesauce, cnd, swtnd, wo/ salt (includes usda commodity)	1 cup	68	0.16	0.17	17.49	1.2	2	0	3	0	0.12	75
applesauce, cnd, unswtnd, wo/added vit c (includes usda commod)	1 cup	42	0.17	0.1	11.27	1.1	2	0	4	0	0.23	74
apricots, raw	1 cup, halves	48	1.4	0.39	11.12	2	1	0	13	0	0.39	259
arrowhead, raw	1 large	99	5.33	0.29	20.23		22	0	10	0	2.57	922
artichokes, (globe or french), ckd, bld, drnd, wo/salt	1 artichoke	53	2.89	0.34	11.95	5.7	60	0	21	0	0.61	286
artichokes, (globe or french), raw	1 artichoke	47	3.27	0.15	10.51	5.4	94	0	44	0	1.28	370
artificial blueberry muffin mix, dry	1 muffin	407	4.7	8.7	77.45		760					
arugula, raw	1 leaf	25	2.58	0.66	3.65	1.6	27	0	160	0	1.46	369
asparagus, ckd, bld, drnd	.5 cup	22	2.4	0.22	4.11	2	14	0	23	0	0.91	224
asparagus, raw	1 cup	20	2.2	0.12	3.88	2.1	2	0	24	0	2.14	202
avocados, raw, all comm var	1 cup, cubes	160	2	14.66	8.53	6.7	7	0	12	0	0.55	485
bacon, pre-sliced, reduced/low na, unprep	1 slice	407	12.53	39.27	0.83	0	470		4		0.42	506
bacon, turkey, lo na	1 slice	253	13.33	20	4.8	0	900	100	10	10	0.72	156
bagel chips, pln	1 oz	451	12.34	15.14	66.36	4.1	233	0	24	0	5.05	140
bagel, pln, tstd, enr w/ca prop (include onion, poppy, sesame)	1 bagel	264	10.56	1.32	52.38	1.6	422	0	219	0	3.57	107
bagel, w/ brkfst steak, egg, chs, & condmnt	1 bagel	282	15.95	14.07	22.99	0.2	642	130	93	15	2.06	145
bagel, w/ egg, sausage patty, chs, & condmnt	1 bagel	295	12.98	16.97	22.64	0.2	550	133	94	18	1.77	123
bagels, cinnamon-raisin	1 mini bagel	274	9.8	1.7	55.2	2.3	344	0	19	0	3.8	148
bagels, egg	1 oz	278	10.6	2.1	53	2.3	505	24	13		3.98	68
bagels, multigrain	1 bagel	241	9.9	1.24	47.47	6.2	359	6	124	0	2.23	204
bagels, oat bran	1 mini bagel	255	10.7	1.2	53.3	3.6	590	0	12	0	3.08	115
bagels, pln, enr, w/ ca prop (includes onion, poppy, sesame), tstd	1 mini bagel	287	11.14	1.43	57.39	1.8	457	0	15	0	4.5	116
bagels, wheat	1 bagel	250	10.2	1.53	48.89	4.1	439	0	20	0	2.76	165
bagels, whl grain white	.5 bagel	255	9.3	0	54.52	4.7	372	0	93	0	4.19	176
baking chocolate, unsweetened, squares	1 oz	642	14.32	52.31	28.42	16.6	24	2	101	0	17.4	830
bamboo shoots, ckd, bld, drnd, wo/salt	1 cup	12	1.53	0.22	1.92	1	4	0	12	0	0.24	533
banana chips	1 oz	519	2.3	33.6	58.4	7.7	6	0	18	0	1.25	536

Food	Serving	Cals	Protein (g)	Fat (g)	Carbs (g)	Fiber (g)	Sodium (mg)	Cholesterol (mg)	Calcium (mg)	Vit D (IU)	Iron (mg)	Potassium (mg)
bananas, raw	1 cup, mashed	89	1.09	0.33	22.84	2.6	1	0	5	0	0.26	358
barley flour or meal	1 cup	345	10.5	1.6	74.52	10.1	4	0	32	0	2.68	309
basil, fresh	5 leaves	23	3.15	0.64	2.65	1.6	4	0	177	0	3.17	295
bass, freshwater, mxd sp, ckd, dry heat	1 fillet	146	24.18	4.73	0	0	90	87	103		1.91	456
bass, striped, ckd, dry heat	1 fillet	124	22.73	2.99	0	0	88	103	19		1.08	328
beans, baked, home prepared	1 cup	155	5.54	5.15	21.63	5.5	422	5	61	0	1.99	358
beans, bkd, cnd, no salt added	1 cup	105	4.8	0.4	20.49	5.5	1	0	50	0	0.29	296
beans, bkd, cnd, w/franks	1 cup	142	6.75	6.57	15.39	6.9	430	6	48	0	1.73	235
beans, bkd, cnd, w/pork	1 cup	106	5.19	1.55	19.99	5.5	414	7	53	0	1.7	309
beans, black, mature ckd, bld, wo/salt	1 cup	132	8.86	0.54	23.71	8.7	1	0	27	0	2.1	355
beans, chili, barbecue, ranch style, ckd	1 cup	97	5	1	16.9	4.2	725	0	31	0	1.86	450
beans, cranberry (roman), mature ckd, bld, wo/salt	1 cup	136	9.34	0.46	24.46	8.6	1	0	50	0	2.09	387
beans, cranberry (roman), mature cnd	1 cup	83	5.54	0.28	15.12	6.3	332	0	34	0	1.55	260
beans, kidney, all types, mature ckd, bld, wo/salt	1 cup	127	8.67	0.5	22.8	6.4	1	0	35	0	2.22	405
beans, kidney, all types, mature cnd	1 cup	84	5.22	0.6	14.5	4.3	296	0	34	0	1.17	237
beans, pinto, cnd, drnd sol	1 can	114	6.99	0.9	20.22	5.5	239	0	63	0	1.33	274
beans, sml white, mature ckd, bld, wo/salt	1 cup	142	8.97	0.64	25.81	10.4	2	0	73	0	2.84	463
beans, snap, cnd, all styles, seasoned, sol&liquids	.5 cup	16	0.83	0.2	3.49	1.5	373	0	22	0	0.47	93
beans, snap, green, raw	1 cup	31	1.83	0.22	6.97	2.7	6	0	37	0	1.03	211
beans, white, mature ckd, bld, wo/salt	1 cup	139	9.73	0.35	25.09	6.3	6	0	90	0	3.7	561
beans, white, mature cnd	1 cup	114	7.26	0.29	21.2	4.8	340	0	73	0	2.99	454
beef jerky, chopd&formed	1 oz	410	33.2	25.6	11	1.8	2081	48	20	11	5.42	597
beef pot pie, frz entree, prep	1 pie	220	7.25	11.39	22.05	0.8	365	21	14		1.25	115
beef sausage, frsh, ckd	1 link	332	18.21	27.98	0.35	0	813	82	11	18	1.57	258
beef stew, canned entree	1 cup	99	4.41	5.53	7.85	0.9	388	13	12	0	2.48	163
beef stks, smoked	1 oz	550	21.5	49.6	5.4		1531	133	68		3.4	257
beef, bologna, red na	1 cup, pieces	310	11.7	28.4	2	0	682	56	12	28	1.4	155
beef, bottom round, roast, lean only, 0" fat, choice, roasted	3 oz	185	27.23	7.63	0	0	36	78	6		2.4	222
beef, brisket, flat half, ln & fat, 0" fat, choic, ckd, brsd	3 oz	221	32.21	9.24	0	0	52	92	17		2.75	254
beef, corned bf hash, w/ potato, cnd	1 cup	164	8.73	10.24	9.27	1.1	412	32	19	0	1	172
beef, cured, brkfst strips, ckd	3 slices	449	31.3	34.4	1.4	0	2253	119	9	7	3.14	412
beef, cured, dried	10 slices	153	31.1	1.94	2.76	0	2790	79	8	1	2.42	235
beef, cured, pastrami	2.5 oz	147	21.8	5.82	0.36	0	1078	68	10	4	2.22	210
beef, cured, sausage, ckd, smoked	1 link	312	14.11	26.91	2.42	0	1131	67	7		1.76	176
beef, ground, 70% ln meat / 30% fat, crumbles, ckd, pan-browned	3 oz	270	25.56	17.86	0	0	96	89	41	2	2.48	328
beef, ground, 80% ln meat / 20% fat, crumbles, ckd, pan-browned	3 oz	272	27	17.36	0	0	91	89	28	2	2.78	380
beef, ground, 90% ln meat / 10% fat, crumbles, ckd, pan-browned	3 oz	230	28.45	12.04	0	0	87	89	16	2	3.08	433
beef, ground, 97% ln meat / 3% fat, crumbles, ckd, pan-browned	3 oz	175	29.46	5.46	0	0	84	89	7	2	3.29	470
beef, ground, unspec fat content, ckd	3 oz	240	25.07	14.53	0.62	0	85	84	25	8	2.67	353
beef, rib, shortribs, ln, choic, ckd, brsd	1 rib	295	30.76	18.13	0	0	58	93	11	12	3.36	313
beef, shldr pot rst, bnless, ln & fat, 0" fat, all grds, ckd, brsd	3 oz	204	31.03	8.92	0	0	61	98	13	6	3.53	352
beef, shldr top blade steak, bnless, ln, 0" fat, all grds, ckd, gri	3 oz	196	28.15	9.23	0	0	87	95	14	5	3.14	390
beef, shoulder steak, boneless, lean only, 0", choice, grill	3 oz	178	28.54	6.25	0	0	68	81	12	5	2.95	372
beef, tenderloin, rst, ln & fat, 1/8" fat, all grds, ckd, rstd	3 oz	324	23.9	24.6	0	0	57	85	9		3.11	331
beer, lt	1 fl oz	29	0.24	0	1.64	0	4	0	4	0	0.03	21
beer, lt, lo carb	1 fl oz	27	0.17	0	0.73	0	3	0	4	0	0	17
beer, reg, all	1 fl oz	43	0.46	0	3.55	0	4	0	4	0	0.02	27
beets, ckd, bld, drnd	.5 cup	44	1.68	0.18	9.96	2	77	0	16	0	0.79	305
beets, raw	1 cup	43	1.61	0.17	9.56	2.8	78	0	16	0	0.8	325

197

Food	Serving	Cals	Protein (g)	Fat (g)	Carbs (g)	Fiber (g)	Sodium (mg)	Cholesterol (mg)	Calcium (mg)	Vit D (IU)	Iron (mg)	Potassium (mg)
biscuit	1 biscuit	370	7.08	18.92	42.82	2.5	979	2	70	0	2.76	131
biscuit w/ egg	1 biscuit	274	8.53	16.23	23.46	0.6	655	180	60		2.13	175
biscuit w/ egg & steak	1 biscuit	277	12.12	19.21	14.37		600	184	93		3.58	207
biscuit, w/ crispy chick fillet	1 biscuit	300	11.93	14.93	30.56	1.4	868	24	44	4	1.76	206
biscuit, w/egg, chs, &bacon	1 biscuit	301	12.01	17.48	24.44	0.2	816	166	103	21	1.57	131
biscuit, w/egg&bacon	1 biscuit	305	11.33	20.73	19.06	0.5	844	235	126	25	2.49	167
biscuit, w/egg&ham	1 biscuit	233	10.64	14.08	16.37	0.4	1093	156	115	25	2.37	166
biscuit, w/ham	1 biscuit	342	11.85	16.3	38.75	0.7	974	22	142	13	2.41	174
biscuit, w/sausage	1 biscuit	371	9.67	24.42	29.99	0.4	814	28	47	14	1.86	153
biscuits, pln or bttrmlk, dry mix, prep	1 oz	335	7.3	12.1	48.4	1.8	955	4	185		2.05	188
biscuits, pln or bttrmlk, frz, bkd	1 oz	338	6.2	11.03	53.87	1.3	942	1	49	0	3.3	224
biscuits, pln or bttrmlk, prep from recipe	1 oz	353	7	16.3	44.6	1.5	580	3	235		2.9	121
bison, ground, grass-fed, ckd	3 oz	179	25.45	8.62	0	0	76	71	14	0	3.19	353
blackberries, frz, unswtnd	1 cup	64	1.18	0.43	15.67	5	1	0	29	0	0.8	140
blackberries, raw	1 cup	43	1.39	0.49	9.61	5.3	1	0	29	0	0.62	162
blueberries, frz, unswtnd	1 cup	51	0.42	0.32	12.17	2.7	1	0	8	0	0.18	54
blueberries, raw	1 cup	57	0.74	0.33	14.49	2.4	1	0	6	0	0.28	77
bologna, meat & poultry	1 slice	281	10.34	23.77	6.31	0	1379	92	125	34	1.24	320
bologna, pork	1 slice	247	15.3	19.87	0.73	0	907	59	11	56	0.77	281
brazil nuts, dried, unblanched	1 cup	659	14.32	67.1	11.74	7.5	3	0	160	0	2.43	659
brd, gluten-free, white, made w/ tapioca starch & brwn rice flr	1 slice	298	5.4	8.02	51.15	5.5	515		59		0.51	107
bread sticks, plain	1 oz	412	12	9.5	68.4	3	713	0	22	0	4.28	124
bread stuffing, bread, dry mix, prep	1 oz	195	2.73	12.05	18.84	0.8	479	0	30	0	0.95	67
bread, banana, prep from recipe, made w/margarine	1 oz	326	4.3	10.5	54.6	1.1	302	43	21		1.4	134
bread, cornbread, dry mix, prep w/ 2% milk, 80% margarine, & eggs	1 muffin	330	6.59	9.58	54.46	2.3	599	57	135	0	1.85	133
bread, cornbread, prep from recipe, made w/lofat (2%) milk	1 oz	266	6.7	7.1	43.5		658	40	249		2.5	147
bread, cracked-wheat	1 oz	260	8.7	3.9	49.5	5.5	538	0	43		2.81	177
bread, egg	1 oz	287	9.5	6	47.8	2.3	380	51	93	16	3.04	115
bread, french	1 oz	272	10.75	2.42	51.88	2.2	602	0	52	0	3.91	117
bread, italian	1 oz	271	8.8	3.5	50.1	3.2	550	0	78	0	2.94	110
bread, multi-grain (includes whole-grain)	1 oz	265	13.36	4.23	43.34	7.4	381	0	103	0	2.5	230
bread, naan, pln, commly prep, refr	1 piece	291	9.62	5.65	50.43	2.2	465		84		3.25	125
bread, oat bran	1 oz	236	10.4	4.4	39.8	4.5	353	0	65	0	3.12	147
bread, oatmeal	1 oz	269	8.4	4.4	48.5	4	447	0	66	0	2.7	142
bread, pan dulce, swt yeast bread	1 slice	367	9.42	11.58	56.38	2.3	228	30	86	0	2.87	103
bread, pita, whole-wheat	1 pita	262	9.8	1.71	55.89	6.1	527	0	15	0	3.06	170
bread, potato	1 slice	266	12.5	3.13	47.07	6.3	375	0	188	2	2.25	718
bread, pound cake type, pan de torta salvadoran	100 g	390	7.06	17.45	51.29	1.7	390		46		2.2	210
bread, pumpernickel	1 oz	250	8.7	3.1	47.5	6.5	596	0	68	0	2.87	208
bread, rye	1 oz	259	8.5	3.3	48.3	5.8	603	0	73	0	2.83	166
bread, wheat	1 slice	274	10.67	4.53	47.54	4	473	0	125	0	3.6	141
bread, wheat, tstd	1 oz	313	12.96	4.27	55.77	4.7	601	0	165	0	4.09	223
bread, whole-wheat, comm. prepared	1 slice	252	12.45	3.5	42.71	6	455	0	161	0	2.47	254
breadnut tree dried	1 cup	367	8.62	1.68	79.39	14.9	53	0	94	0	4.6	2011
breadnut tree raw	1 oz	217	5.97	0.99	46.28		31	0	98	0	2.09	1183
breadstick, soft, prep w/ garlic & parmesan chs	1 breadstick	343	12.2	12.88	44.48	2.4	539	7	87	2	4.65	132
breakfast burrito, w/ egg, chs, & sausage	1 burrito	277	11.1	15.63	22.97	1.2	744	137	132	31	2.28	150
breakfast items, biscuit w/ egg&sausage	1 biscuit	312	11.13	20.77	21.05	0.2	672	161	51	22	1.9	149
broccoli raab, ckd	1 cup	33	3.83	0.52	3.12	2.8	56	0	118	0	1.27	343
broccoli raab, raw	1 cup, chopped	22	3.17	0.49	2.85	2.7	33	0	108	0	2.14	196
brussels sprouts, ckd, bld, drnd, wo/salt	1 sprout	36	2.55	0.5	7.1	2.6	21	0	36	0	1.2	317
brussels sprouts, raw	1 cup	43	3.38	0.3	8.95	3.8	25	0	42	0	1.4	389

Food	Serving	Cals	Protein (g)	Fat (g)	Carbs (g)	Fiber (g)	Sodium (mg)	Cholesterol (mg)	Calcium (mg)	Vit D (IU)	Iron (mg)	Potassium (mg)
buckwheat	1 cup	343	13.25	3.4	71.5	10	1	0	18	0	2.2	460
buckwheat flr, whole-groat	1 cup	335	12.62	3.1	70.59	10	11	0	41	0	4.06	577
burrito, bean and cheese, frozen	1 burrito	221	7.07	6.3	34.01	3.4	351	2	52	0	2.51	210
burrito, w/ bns & bf	1 burrito	191	11.52	7.47	19.52	3	570	26	90	3	1.91	269
burrito, w/bns	2 pieces	206	6.48	6.22	32.92		454	2	52		2.08	301
burrito, w/bns, chs, &bf	1 burrito	180	7.03	6.8	23.37	3.7	451	12	90	3	1.82	204
burrito, w/bns&chs	1 burrito	205	7.35	6.05	31.23	4.2	563	5	124	2	2.37	261
butter oil, anhydrous	1 tbsp	876	0.28	99.48	0	0	2	256	4	0	0	5
butter replcmnt, wo/fat, pdr	1 cup	373	2	1	89	0	1200	2	23	0	2	2
butter, with salt	1 pat	717	0.85	81.11	0.06	0	643	215	24	0	0.02	24
butter, without salt	1 pat	717	0.85	81.11	0.06	0	11	215	24	0	0.02	24
butterscotch	1 oz	391	0.03	3.3	90.4	0	391	9	4	0	0.01	3
cabbage, ckd, bld, drnd, wo/salt	.5 cup, shredded	23	1.27	0.06	5.51	1.9	8	0	48	0	0.17	196
cabbage, raw	1 cup, chopped	25	1.28	0.1	5.8	2.5	18	0	40	0	0.47	170
cake, angelfood, commly prep	1 oz	258	5.9	0.8	57.8	1.5	749	0	140		0.52	93
cake, angelfood, dry mix, prep	1 oz	257	6.1	0.3	58.7	0.2	511	0	84	0	0.23	135
cake, boston crm pie, commly prep	1 oz	252	2.4	8.5	42.9	1.4	254	37	23	5	0.38	39
cake, cherry fudge w/choc frstng	1 oz	264	2.4	12.5	38	0.5	164	42	48	14	1.1	166
cake, choc, commly prep w/ choc frstng, in-store bakery	1 oz	389	3.48	20.05	52.84	2.2	348	22	30	0	3.04	270
cake, choc, prep from recipe wo/frstng	1 oz	371	5.3	15.1	53.4	1.6	315	58	60		1.61	140
cake, fruitcake, commly prep	1 oz	324	2.9	9.1	61.6	3.7	101	5	33	0	2.07	153
cake, gingerbread, prep from recipe	1 oz	356	3.9	16.4	49.2		327	32	71		2.88	439
cake, pnappl upside-down, prep from recipe	1 oz	319	3.5	12.1	50.5	0.8	319	22	120		1.48	112
cake, pound, commly prep, butter (includes frsh & frozen)	1/6 loaf	353	5	13.96	53.64	0.6	377	66	47	34	1.48	149
cake, pound, commly prep, fat-free	1 oz	283	5.4	1.2	61	1.1	341	0	43	0	2.06	110
cake, pound, commly prep, other than all butter, enr	1 oz	389	5.2	17.9	52.5	1	400	58	64		1.62	106
cake, shortcake, biscuit-type, prep from recipe	1 oz	346	6.1	14.2	48.5		506	3	205		2.54	106
cake, snack cakes, creme-filled, choc w/ frstng	1 oz	399	3.63	15.93	60.31	3.2	332	0	116	0	3.6	176
cake, snack cakes, creme-filled, sponge	1 oz	374	3.47	11.54	64.03	1	470	41	24	4	1.36	71
cake, sponge, commly prep	1 oz	290	5.4	2.7	61	0.5	623	102	70	9	2.72	99
cake, sponge, prep from recipe	1 oz	297	7.3	4.3	57.7		228	170	42		1.58	141
cake, white, prep from recipe w/ cocnt frstng	1 oz	356	4.4	10.3	63.2	1	284	1	90	8	1.16	99
cake, white, prep from recipe wo/frstng	1 oz	357	5.4	12.4	57.2	0.8	327	2	130		1.52	95
cake, yel, commly prep, w/ choc frstng, in-store bakery	1 oz	379	3.16	17.75	55.36	1.5	310	16	32	6	2.03	187
cake, yel, commly prep, w/vanilla frstng	1 oz	391	2.99	17.91	56.2	0.3	269	75	62	16	1.07	53
cake, yel, prep from recipe wo/frstng	1 oz	361	5.3	14.6	53	0.7	343	54	146		1.64	91
canada goose, breast meat, skinless, raw	3 oz	133	24.31	4.02	0	0	50	80	4		5.91	336
canadian bacon, ckd, pan-fried	1 slice	146	28.31	2.78	1.8	0	993	67	7	9	0.56	999
candied fruit	1 piece	322	0.34	0.07	82.74	1.6	98	0	18	0	0.17	56
candies, hard	1 oz	394	0	0.2	98	0	38	0	3	0	0.3	5
candies, hard, dietetic or lo cal (sorbitol)	1 candy	394	0	0	98.6	0	0	0	0	0	0	0
candies, jellies	1 tbsp	266	0.15	0.02	69.95	1	30	0	7	0	0.19	54
candies, jellies, no sugar (with na saccharin), any flavors	1 cup	121	0.55	0	29.6	2.2	3	0	31	0	0.15	96
capers, canned	1 tbsp, drained	23	2.36	0.86	4.89	3.2	2348	0	40	0	1.67	40
carambola, (starfruit), raw	1 cup, cubes	31	1.04	0.33	6.73	2.8	2	0	3	0	0.08	133
caramels	2.5 oz	382	4.6	8.1	77	0	245	7	138	0	0.14	214
caramels, chocolate-flavor roll	1 piece	387	1.59	3.31	87.73	0.1	44	2	36	0	0.8	116
carb, cola, wo/ caffeine	1 fl oz	41	0	0	10.58	0	4	0	2	0	0.02	3

Food	Serving	Cals	Protein (g)	Fat (g)	Carbs (g)	Fiber (g)	Sodium (mg)	Cholesterol (mg)	Calcium (mg)	Vit D (IU)	Iron (mg)	Potassium (mg)
carob-flavor bev mix, pdr	1 tbsp	372	1.8	0.2	93.3	8	103	0	32		4.6	104
carob-flavor bev mix, pdr, prep w/ whl milk	1 cup	75	3.16	3.11	8.68	0.4	46	10	98		0.25	131
carrot juice, canned	1 cup	40	0.95	0.15	9.28	0.8	66	0	24	0	0.46	292
carrots, baby, raw	1 large carrot	35	0.64	0.13	8.24	2.9	78	0	32	0	0.89	237
carrots, ckd, bld, drnd, wo/salt	1 tbsp	35	0.76	0.18	8.22	3	58	0	30	0	0.34	235
carrots, raw	1 cup, chopped	41	0.93	0.24	9.58	2.8	69	0	33	0	0.3	320
cashew butter, pln, wo/salt	1 tbsp	587	17.56	49.41	27.57	2	15	0	43	0	5.03	546
cashew dry rstd, w/salt	1 cup	574	15.31	46.35	32.69	3	640	0	45	0	6	565
cashew dry rstd, wo/salt	1 cup	574	15.31	46.35	32.69	3	16	0	45	0	6	565
cashew raw	1 oz	553	18.22	43.85	30.19	3.3	12	0	37	0	6.68	660
catchannel, ckd, breaded&fried	1 fillet	229	18.09	13.33	8.04	0.7	280	71	44		1.43	340
catchannel, farmed, ckd, dry heat	1 fillet	144	18.44	7.19	0	0	119	66	9	10	0.28	366
catchannel, farmed, raw	3 oz	119	15.23	5.94	0	0	98	55	8	9	0.23	302
catchannel, wild, ckd, dry heat	1 fillet	105	18.47	2.85	0	0	50	72	11		0.35	419
catchannel, wild, raw	3 oz	95	16.38	2.82	0	0	43	58	14	500	0.3	358
cauliflower, ckd, bld, drnd, wo/salt	.5 cup	23	1.84	0.45	4.11	2.3	15	0	16	0	0.32	142
cauliflower, raw	1 cup, chopped	25	1.92	0.28	4.97	2	30	0	22	0	0.42	299
caviar, black&red, granular	1 tbsp	264	24.6	17.9	4	0	1500	588	275	117	11.88	181
celery, raw	1 cup, chopped	16	0.69	0.17	2.97	1.6	80	0	40	0	0.2	260
chard, swiss, ckd, bld, drnd, wo/salt	1 cup, chopped	20	1.88	0.08	4.13	2.1	179	0	58	0	2.26	549
chard, swiss, raw	1 cup	19	1.8	0.2	3.74	1.6	213	0	51	0	1.8	379
chckn, brolr or fryrs, brst, sknlss, bnless, meat only, ckd, grilld	3 oz	151	30.54	3.17	0	0	52	104	5	1	0.45	391
cheesburger; dbl, rg ptty; dbl bn w/ cndmnt & spl sau	1 sandwich	261	11.94	14.1	21.53	1.4	485	36	127	5	1.4	182
cheesburger; single, lrg patty; w/ condmnt, veg & ham	1 sandwich	286	15.55	18.97	13.01	0	674	48	119		1.98	212
cheese fd, cold pk, american	1 oz	331	19.66	24.46	8.32	0	966	64	497		0.84	363
cheese, american, nonfat or fat free	1 oz	126	21.05	0	10.53	0	1316	26	789	5	0	393
cheese, blue	1 oz	353	21.4	28.74	2.34	0	1146	75	528	21	0.31	256
cheese, brick	1 cup, diced	371	23.24	29.68	2.79	0	560	94	674	22	0.43	136
cheese, brie	1 oz	334	20.75	27.68	0.45	0	629	100	184	20	0.5	152
cheese, camembert	1 oz	300	19.8	24.26	0.46	0	842	72	388	18	0.33	187
cheese, caraway	1 oz	376	25.18	29.2	3.06	0	690	93	673		0.64	93
cheese, cheddar	1 cup, diced	404	22.87	33.31	3.09	0	653	99	710	24	0.14	76
cheese, cheddar, nonfat or fat free	1 oz	157	32.14	0	7.14	0	1000	18	893	5	0	66
cheese, cheddar, red fat	1 slice	309	27.35	20.41	4.06	0	628	76	761	13	0.12	63
cheese, cheddar, sharp, sliced	1 slice	410	24.25	33.82	2.13	0	644	99	711	41	0.16	76
cheese, cheshire	1 oz	387	23.37	30.6	4.78	0	700	103	643		0.21	95
cheese, colby	1 cup, diced	394	23.76	32.11	2.57	0	604	95	685	24	0.76	127
cheese, cottage, crmd, lrg or sml curd	4 oz	98	11.12	4.3	3.38	0	364	17	83	3	0.07	104
cheese, cottage, nonfat, uncrmd, dry, lrg or sml curd	1 cup	72	10.34	0.29	6.66	0	372	7	86	0	0.15	137
cheese, cream	1 tbsp	350	6.15	34.44	5.52	0	314	101	97	0	0.11	132
cheese, cream, fat free	1 tbsp	105	15.69	1	7.66	0	702	12	351	0	0.19	278
cheese, cream, low fat	1 tbsp	201	7.85	15.28	8.13	0	359	54	148	11	0.17	247
cheese, edam	1 oz	357	24.99	27.8	1.43	0	812	89	731	20	0.44	188
cheese, feta	1 cup, crumbled	264	14.21	21.28	4.09	0	917	89	493	16	0.65	62
cheese, fontina	1 cup, diced	389	25.6	31.14	1.55	0	800	116	550	23	0.23	64
cheese, goat, semisoft type	1 oz	364	21.58	29.84	0.12	0	415	79	298	22	1.62	158
cheese, gouda	1 oz	356	24.94	27.44	2.22	0	819	114	700	20	0.24	121
cheese, gruyere	1 oz	413	29.81	32.34	0.36	0	714	110	1011	24	0.17	81
cheese, limburger	1 cup	327	20.05	27.25	0.49	0	800	90	497	20	0.13	128
cheese, lofat, cheddar or colby	1 cup, diced	173	24.35	7	1.91	0	873	21	415	5	0.42	66
cheese, mexican blend	.25 cup, shredded	358	23.54	28.51	1.75	0	338	95	659	21	0.59	85
cheese, monterey	1 cup, diced	373	24.48	30.28	0.68	0	600	89	746	22	0.72	81

Food	Serving	Cals	Protein (g)	Fat (g)	Carbs (g)	Fiber (g)	Sodium (mg)	Cholesterol (mg)	Calcium (mg)	Vit D (IU)	Iron (mg)	Potassium (mg)
cheese, mozzarella, non-fat	1 cup, shredded	141	31.7	0	3.5	1.8	743	18	961	0	0.31	106
cheese, mozzarella, part skim milk	1 oz	254	24.26	15.92	2.77	0	619	64	782	12	0.22	84
cheese, mozzarella, whl milk	1 cup, shredded	300	22.17	22.35	2.19	0	627	79	505	16	0.44	76
cheese, muenster	1 cup, diced	368	23.41	30.04	1.12	0	628	96	717	22	0.41	134
cheese, muenster, low fat	1 cup, shredded	271	24.7	17.6	3.5	0	600	63	529	13	0.41	134
cheese, neufchatel	1 oz	253	9.15	22.78	3.59	0	334	74	117		0.13	152
cheese, parmesan, dry grated, red fat	1 cup	265	20	20	1.37	0	1529	88	1109	15	0.9	125
cheese, parmesan, grated	1 cup	420	28.42	27.84	13.91	0	1804	86	853	21	0.49	180
cheese, parmesan, hard	1 oz	392	35.75	25.83	3.22	0	1376	68	1184	19	0.82	92
cheese, parmesan, shredded	1 tbsp	415	37.86	27.34	3.41	0	1696	72	1253	21	0.87	97
cheese, provolone	1 cup, diced	351	25.58	26.62	2.14	0	876	69	756	20	0.52	138
cheese, ricotta, whole milk	.5 cup	174	11.26	12.98	3.04	0	84	51	207	10	0.38	105
cheese, romano	1 oz	387	31.8	26.94	3.63	0	1433	104	1064	20	0.77	86
cheese, roquefort	1 oz	369	21.54	30.64	2	0	1809	90	662		0.56	91
cheese, swiss	1 cup, diced	393	26.96	30.99	1.44	0	187	93	890	0	0.13	72
cheese, white, queso blanco	1 cup, crumbled	310	20.38	24.31	2.53		704	70	690	27	0.18	126
cheeseburger; double, reg patty & bun, w/ condmnt	1 sandwich	282	16.24	16.18	17.97	1	617	50	150	7	2.35	226
cheeseburger; dble, reg, patty & bn; w/ condmnt & veg	1 sandwich	285	13.04	15.47	23.3		404	41	74		2.07	171
cheeseburger; double; lrg patty, w/ condmnt & veg	1 sandwich	273	14.72	16.92	15.37		445	55	93		2.29	231
cheeseburger; double; lrg patty; w/ condmnt	1 sandwich	272	16.96	16.22	14.43	1	480	57	106		2.18	242
cheeseburger; double; lrg patty; w/ condmnt, veg & mayo	1 sandwich	253	15.5	15.63	12.62	1.3	405	49	68	4	4.12	202
cheeseburger; double, reg patty, w/ condmnt & veg	1 sandwich	251	12.8	12.7	21.2		633	36	103		2.06	202
cheeseburger; double, reg patty; pln	1 sandwich	308	17.16	17.4	20.8	0.7	621	55	180		2.37	216
cheeseburger; double; reg patty; w/ condmnt	1 sandwich	282	16.24	16.18	17.97	0.9	617	50	150	7	2.35	226
cheeseburger; single, lrg patty; pln	1 sandwich	310	17.29	15.97	24.07	1.7	481	51	114	2	2.57	210
cheeseburger; single, lrg patty; w/ condmnt	1 sandwich	269	15.21	14.4	19.72	1.2	591	48	179	3	1.02	223
cheeseburger; single, lrg patty; w/ condmnt & veg	1 sandwich	206	11.59	10.36	16.81	1.4	385	34	95		1.86	210
cheeseburger; single, reg patty, w/ condmnt	1 sandwich	270	13.49	12.9	25.46	1.9	628	39	123	3	2.25	184
cheeseburger; single, reg patty, w/ condmnt & veg	1 sandwich	254	13.06	11.5	24.97	1.4	546	36	92	2	2.78	178
cheeseburger; single, reg patty; pln	1 sandwich	308	16.51	14.72	28.03	2	515	43	119	2	2.71	196
cheeseburger; triple, reg patty; pln	1 sandwich	310	18.2	19.17	16.16	0.5	637	63	174		2.23	230
cheesecake commly prep	1 oz	321	5.5	22.5	25.5	0.4	438	55	51	18	0.63	90
cheesecake prep from mix, no-bake type	1 oz	274	5.5	12.7	35.5	1.9	380	29	172		0.47	211
cherries, sour, red, raw	1 cup, without pits	50	1	0.3	12.18	1.6	3	0	16	0	0.32	173
cherries, sweet, raw	1 cup, with pits yields	63	1.06	0.2	16.01	2.1	0	0	13	0	0.36	222
cherries, tart, dried, swtnd	.25 cup	333	1.25	0.73	80.45	2.5	13	0	38	0	0.68	376
chesebrger; sing, lrg paty; w/ condmnt, veg & mayo	1 sandwich	268	13.69	15.8	17.73	1.1	473	51	73	3	2.3	208
cheseburger; single, lrg patty; w/ condmnt & bacon	1 sandwich	282	15.78	15.86	18.89	1.3	674	50	137		2.07	238
chewing gum	1 stick	360	0	0.3	96.7	2.4	1	0	0	0	0	2
chewing gum, sugarless	1 piece	268	0	0.4	94.8	2.4	7	0	20	0	0	0
chia dried	1 oz	486	16.54	30.74	42.12	34.4	16	0	631		7.72	407
chick tenders	1 strip	271	19.22	13.95	17.25	1.2	769	48	17	7	0.73	373
chicken breast oven-roasted fat-free sliced	2 slices	79	16.79	0.39	2.17	0	1087	36	6		0.32	67

Food	Serving	Cals	Protein (g)	Fat (g)	Carbs (g)	Fiber (g)	Sodium (mg)	Cholesterol (mg)	Calcium (mg)	Vit D (IU)	Iron (mg)	Potassium (mg)
chicken breast tenders, breaded, ckd, microwaved	1 tender	252	16.35	12.89	17.56	0	446	45	14		1	225
chicken breast, deli, rotisserie seasoned, sliced, prepackaged	1 slice	98	17.4	1.86	2.92	0	1032	51	11	2	0.39	360
chicken filet sndwch, w/ lettuce & mayo, crispy	1 sandwich	276	10.94	13.59	27.4	1.4	617	29	72	7	1.71	179
chicken fillet sndwch, pln w/ pickles	1 sandwich	250	16.28	11.19	20.89	1.4	753	35	58	5	1.77	245
chicken in tortilla, w/ lttc, chs, & ranch sau, crispy	1 wrap	275	11.48	15.1	23.22	1.3	607	29	88	4	1.47	173
chicken pot pie, frz entree, prep	1 pie	204	5.11	11.85	19.21	1.1	393	15	20	2	0.76	110
chicken tenders, breaded, frz, prep	1 tender	240	14.62	13.58	14.86	1.7	527	36	39	3	0.84	281
chicken, bacon, & tomato club sndwch, w/ chs, letuce, & mayo, crispy	1 sandwich	257	15.38	11.76	22.61	1.2	605	38	92	7	1.32	256
chicken, breaded & fried, bnless pieces, pln	6 pieces	307	15.92	20.36	14.93	0.9	594	55	11	7	0.83	251
chicken, broiler or fryer, meat&skn&giblets&neck, fried, batter	3 oz	291	22.84	17.53	9.03		284	103	21		1.79	190
chicken, broiler, rotisserie, bbq, drumstk meat & skn	1 drumstick	206	25.65	11.46	0.12	0	392	149	22	0	1.02	283
chicken, broiler, rotisserie, bbq, drumstk, meat only	1 drumstick	172	27.71	6.76	0	0	403	155	20	0	1.05	291
chicken, broiler, rotisserie, bbq, thigh meat & skn	1 thigh	226	22.51	15.08	0.12	0	335	127	16	0	0.95	255
chicken, broiler, rotisserie, bbq, thigh, meat only	1 thigh	193	24.09	10.74	0	0	335	128	13	0	0.97	262
chicken, broiler, rotisserie, bbq, wing meat & skn	1 wing	257	23.42	18.04	0.6	0	579	129	33	0	0.93	285
chicken, broiler, rotisserie, bbq, wing, meat only	1 wing	184	28.34	7.79	0.54	0	725	134	32	0	0.97	322
chicken, broilers or fryers, back, meat & skn, ckd, rotisserie, or	1 back	260	23.23	18.59	0.03	0	584	128	35		0.97	291
chicken, broilers or fryers, back, meat&skn, ckd, fried, flr	1 piece	331	27.79	20.74	6.5		90	89	24		1.62	226
chicken, broilers or fryers, breast, meat only, ckd, fried	1 piece	187	33.44	4.71	0.51	0	79	91	16	5	1.14	276
chicken, broilers or fryers, breast, meat&skn, ckd, fried, batter	1 piece	260	24.84	13.2	8.99	0.3	275	85	20	6	1.25	201
chicken, broilers or fryers, drumstk, meat only, ckd, fried	1 piece	195	28.62	8.08	0	0	96	94	12		1.32	249
chicken, broilers or fryers, drumstk, meat&skn, ckd, fried, batter	1 piece	268	21.95	15.75	8.28	0.3	269	86	17		1.35	186
chicken, nuggets, dk & white meat, preckd, frz, not rehtd	4 nuggets	268	12.02	17.31	16.09	1.6	540	32	47	10	0.95	206
chicken, nuggets, white meat, preckd, frz, not rehtd	4 nuggets	261	14.36	15.42	16.24	0.7	538	34	38		1.43	281
chickpea flour (besan)	1 cup	387	22.39	6.69	57.82	10.8	64	0	45	0	4.86	846
chickpeas , mature ckd, bld, wo/salt	1 cup	164	8.86	2.59	27.42	7.6	7	0	49	0	2.89	291
chili con carne w/bns, cnd entree	1 cup	107	5.8	3.47	13.1	3.3	449	9	33	1	1.34	264
chili powder	1 tsp	282	13.46	14.28	49.7	34.8	2867	0	330	0	17.3	1950
chili w/ bns, microwavable bowls	1 cup	100	5.85	3.68	10.88	2.9	385	10	34	0	1.13	245
chili with beans, canned	1 cup	103	6.12	3.76	13.24	3.3	423	17	47	0	3.43	365
chili, no bns, cnd entree	1 cup	118	7.53	7.1	6.1	0.5	411	21	30	3	2.01	185
chips corn-based, extruded, pln	1 oz	538	6.17	33.36	56.9	4	514	0	138	0	1.2	144
chips, corn-base, extrud, barbecue-flavor, w/enr masa flr	1 oz	523	7	32.7	56.2		763	0	131		4.9	236
chips, corn-based, extruded, onion-flavor	1 oz	499	7.7	22.6	65.1	3.9	950	0	29	0	3.72	143
chives, raw	1 tbsp, chopped	30	3.27	0.73	4.35	2.5	3	0	92	0	1.6	296
choc covered, caramel w/nuts	1 piece	470	9.5	21	60.67	4.3	156	0	78	0	1.7	445
choc malt, pdr, prep w/ fat free milk	3 tbsp	49	3.25	0.17	8.64	0	77	2	234	60	0.74	158
choc syrup	2 tbsp	279	2.1	1.13	65.1	2.6	72	0	14	0	2.11	224
chocolate almond milk, unswtnd, shelf-stable, fort w/ vit d2 & e	1 cup	21	0.83	1.46	1.25	0.4	75	0	188	42	0.45	96

Food	Serving	Cals	Protein (g)	Fat (g)	Carbs (g)	Fiber (g)	Sodium (mg)	Cholesterol (mg)	Calcium (mg)	Vit D (IU)	Iron (mg)	Potassium (mg)
chocolate dairy drk mix, red cal, w/ low-cal sweeteners, pdr	1 packet, (.75 oz)	329	25	2.6	51.4	9.4	659	24	1412	188	7.7	2240
chocolate malt pdr, prep w/ 1% milk, fort	1 cup, dry mix	57	3.32	0.97	8.81	0	60	5	160	100	1.14	191
chocolate pdr, no sugar added	2 tbsp	373	9.09	9.09	63.64	9.1	636	0	909	0	3.27	1705
chocolate syrup, prep w/ whl milk	1 cup	90	3.07	2.96	12.78	0.3	47	9	89		0.32	145
chocolate-fla bev mix , mlk, pdr, w/ add nutr, prep w/ whl milk	1 cup	89	3.27	3.17	11.87	0.4	50	10	141	47	0.03	144
chocolate-flavor bev mix for milk, pdr, w/ added nutr	1 cup	400	4.55	2.27	90.28	4.5	136	0	455	0	0	280
chocolate-flavor bev mix, pdr, prep w/ whl milk	1 cup	85	3.23	3.24	11.91	0.4	58	9	95		0.3	172
chocolate-flavored drk, whey & milk bsd	1 cup	49	0.64	0.4	10.68	0.6	91	0	100	50	0.33	79
chocolate-flavored frstd puffed corn	1 cup	405	3.34	3.5	87.2	3.8	534	0	70	0	15.87	176
chocolate-flavored hazelnut sprd	2 tbsp	541	5.41	29.73	62.16	5.4	41	0	108	0	4.38	407
chocolate, dk, 45- 59% cacao sol	1 oz	546	4.88	31.28	61.17	7	24	8	56		8.02	559
chocolate, dk, 60-69% cacao sol	1 oz	579	6.12	38.31	52.42	8	10	6	62		6.32	567
chocolate, dk, 70-85% cacao sol	1 oz	598	7.79	42.63	45.9	10.9	20	3	73		11.9	715
chocolate, dk, nfs (45-59% cacao sol 90%; 60-69% cacao sol	1 oz	550	5.09	32.2	59.97	7.2	23	7	57	0	8.13	568
choolate dark, milk & soy bsd, ready to drk, fort	8 fl oz	101	4.22	1.69	17.3	1.3	63	4	127	101	1.9	245
cinnamon buns, frstd (includes honey buns)	1 bun	452	4.45	26.61	48.6	1.2	305	5	183	0	1.37	102
cinnamon rolls, mini	1 roll	403	7.02	17.95	53.38	2.2	554	21	54		2.55	131
cinnamon, ground	1 tsp	247	3.99	1.24	80.59	53.1	10	0	1002	0	8.32	431
citrus fruit juc drk, frz conc	1 fl oz	162	1.2	0.1	40.2	0.2	3	0	25	0	3.94	393
citrus fruit juc drk, frz conc, prep w/ h2o	1 fl oz	46	0.34	0.03	11.42	0.1	4	0	9		1.12	112
clam & tomato juc, cnd	1 fl oz	48	0.6	0.2	10.95	0.4	362	0	8		0.15	89
clam, mxd sp, ckd, breaded&fried	3 oz	202	14.24	11.15	10.33		364	61	63		13.91	326
clam, mxd sp, ckd, moist heat	3 oz	148	25.55	1.95	5.13	0	1202	67	92		2.81	628
clementines, raw	1 fruit	47	0.85	0.15	12.02	1.7	1	0	30	0	0.14	177
cloves, ground	1 tsp	274	5.97	13	65.53	33.9	277	0	632	0	11.83	1020
club soda	1 fl oz	0	0	0	0	0	21	0	5	0	0.01	2
cocoa mix, lo cal, pdr, w/ add ca, p, asprt, wo/ add na, vit a	1 envelope	359	25.1	3	58	1.1	653	11	1440	0	4.96	2702
cocktail mix, non-alcoholic, concd, frz	1 fl oz	287	0.08	0.01	71.6	0	0	0	2	0	0.04	23
cocoa mix, no sugar added, pdr	1 envelope	377	15.49	3	71.93	7.5	876	0	576	0	4.96	2702
cocoa mix, pdr	1 envelope	398	6.67	4	83.73	3.7	504	0	133	0	1.19	712
cocoa mix, pdr, prep w/ h2o	1 fl oz	55	0.92	0.55	11.54	0.5	73	0	21		0.17	99
cocoa mix, w/ asprt, pdr, prep w/ h2o	1 fl oz	29	1.21	0.23	5.61	0.6	72	0	48		0.39	211
cocoa, dry pdr, unswtnd	1 cup	228	19.6	13.7	57.9	37	21	0	128	0	13.86	1524
coconut bar, not choc covered	1 bar	481	2.13	27.65	55.87	6.4	128	0	43	0	0.77	294
coconut crm, cnd, swtnd	1 tbsp	357	1.17	16.31	53.21	0.2	36	0	4	0	0.13	101
coconut crm, raw (liq expressed from grated meat)	1 tbsp	330	3.63	34.68	6.65	2.2	4	0	11	0	2.28	325
coconut h2o (liq from coconuts)	1 cup	19	0.72	0.2	3.71	1.1	105	0	24	0	0.29	250
coconut h2o, rtd, unswtnd	1 cup	18	0.22	0	4.24	0	26	0	7	0	0.03	165
coconut meat, raw	1 cup, shredded	354	3.33	33.49	15.23	9	20	0	14	0	2.43	356
coconut milk, swtnd, fort w/ ca, vitamins a, b12, d2	1 cup	31	0.21	2.08	2.92	0	19	0	188	42	0.3	19
cod, atlantic, ckd, dry heat	3 oz	105	22.83	0.86	0	0	78	55	14	46	0.49	244
cod, atlantic, cnd, sol&liq	3 oz	105	22.76	0.86	0	0	218	55	21	47	0.49	528
cod, atlantic, dried&salted	1 oz	290	62.82	2.37	0	0	7027	152	160	161	2.5	1458
cod, pacific, ckd (not previously frozen)	3 oz	84	20.42	0.25	0		134	61	17		0.16	372
cod, pacific, ckd, dry heat (maybe previously frozen)	1 fillet	85	18.73	0.5	0	0	372	57	10	24	0.2	289
coffee sub, crl grain bev, pdr	1 tsp	360	6.01	2.52	78.42	23.3	83	0	58	0	4.6	2443
coffee sub, crl grain bev, pdr, prep w/ whl milk	6 fl oz	65	3.3	3.3	5.6	0.1	49	13	119		0.11	172

Food	Serving	Cals	Protein (g)	Fat (g)	Carbs (g)	Fiber (g)	Sodium (mg)	Cholesterol (mg)	Calcium (mg)	Vit D (IU)	Iron (mg)	Potassium (mg)
coffee sub, crl grain bev, prep w/ h2o	1 fl oz	6	0.1	0.04	1.3	0.4	5	0	4	0	0.08	41
coffee, brewed, brkfst blend	1 cup	2	0.3	0	0.23	0	1	0	2	0	0.02	50
coffee, brewed, espresso, rest-prep	1 fl oz	9	0.12	0.18	1.67	0	14	0	2	0	0.13	115
coffee, brewed, espresso, rest-prep, decaffeinated	1 fl oz	9	0.1	0.18	1.69	0	14	0	2	0	0.13	115
coffee, brewed, prep w/ tap h2o	1 fl oz	1	0.12	0.02	0	0	2	0	2	0	0.01	49
coffee, brewed, prep w/ tap h2o, decaffeinated	1 fl oz	0	0.1	0	0	0	2	0	2	0	0.05	54
coffee, inst, chicory	1 fl oz	3	0.09	0	0.75	0	7	0	4		0.05	35
coffee, inst, decaffeinated, pdr	1 tsp	351	11.6	0.2	76	0	23	0	140	0	3.8	3501
coffee, inst, decaffeinated, prep w/ h2o	1 fl oz	2	0.12	0	0.43	0	4	0	4		0.04	36
coffee, inst, mocha, swtnd	2 tbsp	460	5.29	15.87	74.04	1.9	317	0	271	0	0	1033
coffee, inst, reg, half the caffeine	1 tsp	352	14.42	0.5	73.18	0	37	0	141	0	4.41	3535
coffee, inst, reg, pdr	1 tsp	353	12.2	0.5	75.4	0	37	0	141	0	4.41	3535
coffee, inst, reg, prep w/ h2o	1 fl oz	2	0.1	0	0.34	0	4	0	4		0.04	30
coffee, inst, vanila, swtnd, decaff, w/ non dairy cream	1 tsp	465	0	13.33	86.28	0	333	0	0	0	0	57
coffee, inst, w/ chicory	1 tsp	355	9.3	0.2	78.9	0.5	277	0	103		4.76	3395
coffee, inst, w/ whtnr, red cal	1 tsp, dry	509	1.96	29.1	59.94	0.5	0	0	18	0	0.06	909
coffee, ready to drk, iced, mocha, milk bsd	1 cup	60	1.48	0.98	11.42	0	31	0	52	0	0.09	136
coffee, ready to drk, milk bsd, swtnd	1 cup	71	1.98	1.38	12.6	0	26	5	74	1	0.04	175
coffee, ready to drk, vanilla, lt, milk bsd, swtnd	9.5 fl oz	36	2.14	1.07	4.27	0	34	5	71	1	0	175
coffee & cocoa, inst, decaffeinated, w/ whtnr&localswtnr	1 tsp, dry	440	9	13.21	71.4	4.8	500	0	60	0	3.06	1856
coffeecake, cheese	1 oz	339	7	15.2	44.3	1	339	85	59		0.64	289
cola or peper-type, w/ na saccharin, caffeine, lo cal	1 fl oz	0	0	0	0.1	0	16	0	4		0.02	4
cola or pepper-type, w/ asprt, wo/ caf, lo cal	1 fl oz	1	0.12	0	0.12	0	4	0	3	0	0.02	7
cola, fast-food cola	1 fl oz	37	0.07	0.02	9.56	0	4	0	2	0	0.11	2
cola, reg	1 fl oz	42	0	0.25	10.36	0	3	0	1	0	0.02	5
coleslaw	1 cup	153	0.95	9.91	14.89	1.9	203	4	30		0.22	129
collards, ckd, bld, drnd, wo/salt	1 cup, chopped	33	2.71	0.72	5.65	4	15	0	141	0	1.13	117
collards, frz, chopd, ckd, bld, drnd, wo/salt	1 cup, chopped	36	2.97	0.41	7.1	2.8	50	0	210	0	1.12	251
collards, raw	1 cup, chopped	32	3.02	0.61	5.42	4	17	0	232	0	0.47	213
confectioner's coating, butterscotch	1 cup, chips	539	2.2	29.05	67.1	0	89	0	34	0	0.08	64
confectioner's coating, pnut butter	1 cup, chips	529	18.3	29.8	46.88	5	250	1	110	0	1.7	505
confectioner's coating, yogurt	1 cup, chips	522	5.87	27	63.94	0	88	1	205	0	0.14	290
cookies, brownies, commly prep	1 oz	405	4.8	16.3	63.9	2.1	286	17	29	0	2.25	149
cookies, choc chip sndwch, w/ creme filling	1 cookie	425	2.94	17.65	63.52	0	279	0	0	0	1.06	94
cookies, choc chip, commly prep, soft-type	1 cookie	444	3.63	19.77	65.75	1.8	276		17		4.07	130
cookies, choc chip, prep from recipe, made w/butter	1 oz	488	5.7	28.4	58.2		341	70	38		2.48	221
cookies, choc chip, refr dough, bkd	1 oz	492	4.9	22.6	68.2	1.7	232	27	28		2.5	200
cookies, cocnt macaroon	2 cookies	460	3.02	22.55	61.22	5.1	241	0	5	0	0.82	123
cookies, fig bars	1 oz	348	3.7	7.3	70.9	4.6	350	0	64	0	2.9	207
cookies, fortune	1 oz	378	4.2	2.7	84	1.6	31	2	12	0	1.44	41
cookies, gingersnaps	1 oz	416	5.6	9.8	76.9	2.2	501	0	77	0	6.4	346
cookies, graham crackers, pln or honey (incl cinn)	1 oz	430	6.69	10.6	77.66	3.4	459	0	77	0	3.78	170
cookies, oatmeal sndwch, w/ creme filling	1 cookie	398	2.61	18.29	55.62	2.6	444	0	0	1	1.88	136
cookies, oatmeal, commly prep, reg	1 oz	450	6.2	18.1	68.7	2.8	383	0	37	0	2.58	142
cookies, oatmeal, prep from recipe, w/raisins	1 oz	435	6.5	16.2	68.4		538	33	100		2.65	239
cookies, oatmeal, prep from recipe, wo/raisins	1 oz	447	6.8	17.9	66.4		598	36	105		2.7	182

Food	Serving	Cals	Protein (g)	Fat (g)	Carbs (g)	Fiber (g)	Sodium (mg)	Cholesterol (mg)	Calcium (mg)	Vit D (IU)	Iron (mg)	Potassium (mg)
cookies, pnut butter, prep from recipe	1 oz	475	9	23.8	58.9		518	31	39		2.23	231
cookies, sugar, commly prep, reg (incl vanilla)	1 oz	464	5.35	19.55	67.34	1.3	385	12	35	0	2.24	87
cookies, sugar, prep from recipe, made w/margarine	1 oz	472	5.9	23.4	60	1.2	491	26	73	21	2.33	77
cookies, sugar, refr dough, bkd	1 oz	489	4.7	23.1	65.6	0.9	362	32	90	0	1.84	163
coriander (cilantro) leaves, raw	.25 cup	23	2.13	0.52	3.67	2.8	46	0	67	0	1.77	521
coriander leaf, dried	1 tsp	279	21.93	4.78	52.1	10.4	211	0	1246	0	42.46	4466
corn & rice (includes all brands)	1 cup	378	6.06	1.08	86.85	1.4	795		10		34.06	105
corn dogs, frz, prep	1 corndog	250	8.57	12.02	26.96	1	668	44	72	15	1.9	125
corn-based, extruded, chips, barbecue-flavor	1 oz	523	7	32.7	56.2	5.2	763	0	131		1.54	236
corn-based, extruded, cones, pln	1 oz	510	5.8	26.9	62.9	1.1	1022	0	3		2.54	81
corn-based, extruded, puffs or twists, cheese-flavor	35 pieces	567	5.46	36.54	54.54	0.8	928	7	53	2	1.69	180
corn, swt, white, ckd, bld, drnd, wo/salt	1 ear, small	97	3.34	1.41	21.71	2.7	3	0	2	0	0.55	252
corn, swt, yel, ckd, bld, drnd, wo/salt	1 ear, small	96	3.41	1.5	20.98	2.4	1	0	3	0	0.45	218
cornstarch	1 cup	381	0.26	0.05	91.27	0.9	9	0	2	0	0.47	3
couscous, cooked	1 cup, cooked	112	3.79	0.16	23.22	1.4	5	0	8	0	0.38	58
cowpeas (blackeyes), immat ckd, bld, drnd, wo/ salt	1 cup	97	3.17	0.38	20.32	5	4	0	128	0	1.12	418
cowpeas, catjang, mature ckd, bld, wo/salt	1 cup	117	8.13	0.71	20.32	3.6	19	0	26	0	3.05	375
crab, alaska king, ckd, moist heat	1 leg	97	19.35	1.54	0	0	1072	53	59		0.76	262
crab, alaska king, imitn, made from surimi	3 oz	95	7.62	0.46	15	0.5	529	20	13	0	0.39	90
crab, blue, ckd, moist heat	1 cup, flaked and pieces	83	17.88	0.74	0	0	395	97	91	0	0.5	259
crab, dungeness, ckd, moist heat	3 oz	110	22.32	1.24	0.95	0	378	76	59		0.43	408
crab, queen, ckd, moist heat	3 oz	115	23.72	1.51	0	0	691	71	33		2.88	200
crabapples, raw	1 cup, slices	76	0.4	0.3	19.95		1	0	18		0.36	194
crackers, cheese, regular	.5 oz	489	10.93	22.74	59.42	2.3	973	3	136	1	4.88	156
crackers, chs, sandwich-type w/ chs filling	6 cracker	490	8.92	24.41	58.76	1.9	878	6	89		2.13	295
crackers, chs, sandwich-type w/pnut butter filling	.5 oz	496	12.41	25.12	56.74	3.4	829	0	50	0	2.72	218
crackers, chs, whl grain	55 pieces	412	9.62	16.03	57.29	6.4	802	16	128	3	3.46	212
crackers, flav, fish-shaped	10 goldfish	463	10.16	17.71	65.67	3.1	970		83		4.58	224
crackers, h2o biscuits	4 crackers	384	7.14	7.14	72.81	7.1	571	0	0	0	0	99
crackers, melba toast, pln	.5 oz	390	12.1	3.2	76.6	6.3	598	0	93	0	3.7	202
crackers, multigrain	4 crackers	482	7.1	20.4	67.6	3.5	883	0	14	0	2.59	171
crackers, saltines (incl oyster, soda, soup)	5 crackers	418	9.46	8.64	74.05	2.8	941	0	19	0	5.57	152
crackers, wheat, regular	16 crackers	455	7.3	16.4	70.73	6.9	699	0	92	0	2.64	283
cranberries, dried, swtnd	.25 cup	308	0.17	1.09	82.8	5.3	5	0	9	0	0.39	49
cranberries, raw	1 cup, chopped	46	0.46	0.13	11.97	3.6	2	0	8	0	0.23	80
cranberry juc blend, 100% juc, btld, w/ added vit c & ca	6.75 fl oz	45	0.27	0.12	10.91	0.1	6	0	19	0	0.08	76
cranberry juc cocktail	1 cup	52	0	0.34	12.25		2		3		0.04	19
cranberry juc cocktail, btld	1 fl oz	54	0	0.1	13.52	0	2	0	3	0	0.1	14
cranberry juc cocktail, frz conc, prep w/ h2o	1 fl oz	47	0.01	0	11.81	0	4	0	5		0.07	12
cranberry juc, unswtnd	1 cup	46	0.39	0.13	12.2	0.1	2	0	8	0	0.25	77
cranberry sau, cnd, swtnd	1 cup	159	0.9	0.15	40.4	1.1	5	0	3	0	0.41	28
cranberry-apple juc drk, btld	1 fl oz	63	0	0.11	15.85	0	2	0	3	0	0.07	17
cranberry-apple juc drk, lo cal, w/ vit c added	1 cup	19	0.1	0	4.7	0.1	5	0	10	0	0.06	45
cranberry-apricot juc drk, btld	1 fl oz	64	0.2	0	16.2	0.1	2	0	9		0.15	61
cranberry-grape juc drk, btld	1 fl oz	56	0.2	0.1	14	0.1	3	0	8		0.01	24
craymxd sp, farmed, ckd, moist heat	3 oz	87	17.52	1.3	0	0	97	137	51		1.11	238
cream of wheat, inst, prep w/ h2o, wo/ salt	1 cup	62	1.84	0.24	13.08	0.6	102	0	64		4.96	20

Food	Serving	Cals	Protein (g)	Fat (g)	Carbs (g)	Fiber (g)	Sodium (mg)	Cholesterol (mg)	Calcium (mg)	Vit D (IU)	Iron (mg)	Potassium (mg)
cream, fluid, half and half	1 fl oz	123	3.13	10.39	4.73	0	61	35	107	2	0.05	132
cream, fluid, hvy whipping	1 cup, whipped	340	2.84	36.08	2.74	0	27	113	66	63	0.1	95
cream, fluid, lt (coffee crm or table crm)	1 fl oz	191	2.96	19.1	2.82	0	72	59	91	44	0.05	136
cream, fluid, lt whipping	1 cup, whipped	292	2.17	30.91	2.96	0	34	111	69	23	0.03	97
cream, sour, cultured	1 tbsp	198	2.44	19.35	4.63	0	31	59	101	0	0.07	125
cream, whipped, crm topping, pressurized	1 cup	257	3.2	22.22	12.49	0	8	76	101	16	0.05	147
creamy drsng, made w/sour crm and/or bttrmlk&oil, red cal	1 tbsp	160	1.5	14	7	0	833	0	6	1	0.13	36
creme de menthe, 72 proof	1 fl oz	371	0	0.3	41.6	0	5	0	0	0	0.07	0
crispy bar w/ pnut butter filling	1.5 oz	542	9.53	31.34	55.53	3.3	264	5	70	0	1.3	295
crm of rice, ckd w/h2o, wo/salt	1 cup	52	0.9	0.1	11.4	0.1	1	0	1	0	3.96	20
croissant, w/egg, chs, &bacon	1 sandwich	312	12.58	19.97	20.79	1	602	167	117	31	1.7	156
croissant, w/egg, chs, &ham	1 sandwich	261	12.45	14.95	18.98	0.9	711	140	95	31	1.4	179
croissant, w/egg, chs, &sausage	1 sandwich	308	12.09	21.78	15.9	1.8	577	123	90	27	1.65	158
croissant, w/egg&chs	1 sandwich	304	10.07	19.45	22.45		434	170	192		1.73	137
croissants, butter	1 oz	406	8.2	21	45.8	2.6	467	67	37	0	2.03	118
croutons, plain	.5 oz	407	11.9	6.6	73.5	5.1	698	0	76		4.08	124
croutons, seasoned	.5 oz	465	10.8	18.3	63.5	5	1089	7	96	0	2.82	181
crustaceans, crab, blue, crab cakes, home recipe	1 cake	155	20.21	7.52	0.48	0	330	150	105		1.08	324
crustaceans, shrimp, ckd (not previously frozen)	3 oz	99	23.98	0.28	0.2		111	189	70		0.51	259
cucumber, peeled, raw	1 cup, pared chopped	12	0.59	0.16	2.16	0.7	2	0	14	0	0.22	136
cucumber, with peel, raw	.5 cup, slices	15	0.65	0.11	3.63	0.5	2	0	16	0	0.28	147
curry powder	1 tsp	325	14.29	14.01	55.83	53.2	52	0	525	0	19.1	1170
daiquiri, prepared-from-recipe	1 fl oz	186	0.06	0.06	6.94	0.1	5	0	3		0.09	21
danish pastry, cheese	1 oz	374	8	21.9	37.2	1	417	23	35	2	1.8	98
dessert topping, pdr, 1.5 oz prep w/1/2 cup milk	1 cup	194	3.61	12.72	17.13	0	66	10	90	38	0.04	151
dessert topping, powdered	1.5 oz	577	4.9	39.92	52.54	0	122	0	17	0	0.03	166
dessert topping, pressurized	1 cup	264	0.98	22.3	16.07	0	62	0	5	0	0.02	19
dessert topping, semi solid, frz	1 cup	318	1.25	25.31	23.05	0	25	0	6	0	0.12	18
dip, bean, original flavor	2 tbsp	119	5.44	3.7	15.89	4.9	443	0	26	0	1.6	368
dip, salsa con queso, chs & salsa- med	2 tbsp	143	3.14	9.51	11.14	0.7	796	9	98	0	0.14	105
dk choc coatd coffee bns	28 pieces	540	7.5	30	59.95	7.5	25	13	100		2.7	342
doughcake-type, choc, sugared or glazed	1 oz	417	4.5	19.9	57.4	2.2	215	57	213	0	2.27	106
doughcake-type, pln (includes unsugared, old-fashioned)	1 donut	434	5.31	24.93	47.06	1.7	477	10	40	0	2.53	134
doughcake-type, pln, chocolate-coated or frstd	1 oz	452	4.93	25.25	51.33	1.9	326	19	24	0	4	201
doughcake-type, pln, sugared or glazed	1 oz	426	5.2	22.9	50.8	1.5	402	32	60		1.06	102
doughfrench crullers, glazed	1 oz	412	3.1	18.3	59.5	1.2	345	11	26	0	2.42	78
doughyeast-leavened, glazed, unenr (incl honey buns)	1 oz	403	6.4	22.8	44.3	1.2	342	6	43		0.6	108
doughyeast-leavened, w/creme filling	1 oz	361	6.4	24.5	30	0.8	309	24	25	0	1.83	80
doughyeast-leavened, w/jelly filling	1 oz	340	5.9	18.7	39	0.9	455	26	25	0	1.76	79
dressing, honey mustard, fat-free	2 tbsp	169	1.07	1.47	38.43	1.2	1004	1	24	0	0.36	69
drink mix, dairy, chc, red cal, w/ asprt, pdr, prep w/ h2o & ice	8 fl oz	29	2.19	0.23	4.51	0.8	61	2	127		0.68	197
drum, freshwater, ckd, dry heat	3 oz	153	22.49	6.32	0	0	96	82	77		1.15	353
duck, domesticated, meat only, ckd, rstd	1 cup, chopped or diced	201	23.48	11.2	0	0	65	89	12	4	2.7	252
duck, domesticated, meat&skn, ckd, rstd	1 cup, chopped or diced	337	18.99	28.35	0	0	59	84	11	3	2.7	204
dulce de leche	1 tbsp	315	6.84	7.35	55.35	0	129	29	251	6	0.17	350

Food	Serving	Cals	Protein (g)	Fat (g)	Carbs (g)	Fiber (g)	Sodium (mg)	Cholesterol (mg)	Calcium (mg)	Vit D (IU)	Iron (mg)	Potassium (mg)
dumpling, potato- or cheese-filled, frz	3 pieces	195	5.26	6.14	29.64	0.9	474	4	35	0	1.26	107
edamame, frz, prep	1 cup	121	11.91	5.2	8.91	5.2	6	0	63	0	2.27	436
eel, mxd sp, ckd, dry heat	1 oz, bone-less	236	23.65	14.95	0	0	65	161	26		0.64	349
egg custard, bkd, prepared-from-recipe	.5 cup	104	5.02	4.58	11	0	61	84	107		0.35	148
egg custards, dry mix, prep w/ 2% milk	.5 cup	112	4.13	2.83	17.61	0	87	49	146	44	0.33	214
egg custards, dry mix, prep w/ whl milk	.5 cup	122	3.99	4	17.6	0	84	51	139	47	0.34	207
egg mix, usda cmdty	1 tbsp	555	35.6	34.5	23.97		576	975	171	296	3.23	373
egg rolls, chick, refr, htd	1 roll	197	10.44	4.51	28.54	2.4	478	14	47	1	1.69	281
egg rolls, pork, refr, htd	1 roll	222	9.94	7.17	29.5	2.1	407	14	34	4	1.55	212
egg rolls, veg, frz, prep	1 egg roll	214	5.95	6.97	31.77	2.4	490	0	50	0	1.95	222
egg sub, liq or frz, fat free	.25 cup	48	10	0	2	0	199	0	73	66	1.98	213
egg, scrambled	2 eggs	212	13.84	16.18	2.08	0	187	426	57	46	2.59	147
egg, white, raw, fresh	1 large	52	10.9	0.17	0.73	0	166	0	7	0	0.08	163
egg, whl, ckd, fried	1 large	196	13.61	14.84	0.83	0	207	401	62	88	1.89	152
egg, whl, ckd, hard-boiled	1 cup, chopped	155	12.58	10.61	1.12	0	124	373	50	87	1.19	126
egg, whl, ckd, poached	1 large	143	12.51	9.47	0.71	0	297	370	56	82	1.75	138
egg, whl, ckd, scrmbld	1 large	149	9.99	10.98	1.61	0	145	277	66	72	1.31	132
egg, whole, cooked, omelet	1 tbsp	154	10.57	11.66	0.64	0	155	313	48	69	1.48	117
eggnog	1 cup	88	4.55	4.19	8.05	0	54	59	130	49	0.2	165
eggnog-flavor mix, pdr, prep w/ whl milk	1 cup	95	2.93	3.02	14.2	0	55	11	92		0.12	121
eggplant, ckd, bld, drnd, wo/salt	1 cup	35	0.83	0.23	8.73	2.5	1	0	6	0	0.25	123
eggplant, raw	1 cup, cubes	25	0.98	0.18	5.88	3	2	0	9	0	0.23	229
energy drk w/ carb h2o & hi fructose corn syrup	8 fl oz	62	0.42	0	15	0	48	0	0	0	0	10
energy drk, citrus	8 fl oz	45	0	0	11.27	0	10	0	8	0	0	4
energy drk, sugar free	8 fl oz	4	0.42	0	0.42	0	42	0	0	0	0	0
eng muffin, w/chs&sausage	1 sandwich	338	13.28	20.67	25.28	0.5	668	43	210	17	3.14	179
eng muffin, w/egg, chs, &canadian bacon	1 sandwich	228	13.64	9.66	21.67	0.4	617	168	192	26	2.3	173
eng muffin, w/egg, chs, &sausage	1 sandwich	286	13.38	18.1	17.44	0.2	548	163	168	22	2.63	147
english muffin, pln, enched.w/ca prop (incld sourdough)	1 oz	227	8.87	1.69	44.17	3.5	425	0	163	0	4	109
english muffins, mixed-grain (incl granola)	1 oz	235	9.1	1.8	46.3	2.8	298	0	196	0	3.02	156
english muffins, raisin-cinnamon (includes apple-cinnamon)	1 oz	240	7.91	1.8	48.1	2.6	299	0	114	0	4.5	173
english muffins, wheat	1 oz	223	8.7	2	44.8	4.6	353	0	178	0	2.87	186
english muffins, whole-wheat	1 oz	203	8.8	2.1	40.4	6.7	364	0	265	0	2.45	210
falafel, home-prepared	1 patty	333	13.31	17.8	31.84		294	0	54	0	3.42	585
fat free ice crm, no sugar added, flavors other than choc	.5 cup	129	4.41	0	27.94	7.4	110	0	147	0	0	196
figs, dried, stewed	1 cup	107	1.42	0.4	27.57	4.2	4	0	70	0	0.88	294
figs, dried, uncooked	1 cup	249	3.3	0.93	63.87	9.8	10	0	162	0	2.03	680
fish sndwch, w/tartar sau	1 sandwich	257	10.29	12.45	26.69	1	602	35	37	9	1.5	206
fish sndwch, w/tartar sau&chs	1 sandwich	279	11.26	14.64	26.39	0.8	434	37	120	37	1.56	220
fish stks, frz, prep	1 piece	277	11.01	16.23	21.66	1.5	402	28	16	1	0.84	185
flan, caramel custard, dry mix, prep w/ 2% milk	.5 cup	103	2.99	1.72	18.82	0	113	7	113	36	0.06	163
flan, caramel custard, dry mix, prep w/ whl milk	.5 cup	113	2.95	3	18.68	0	112	12	111	36	0.06	160
flan, caramel custard, prepared-from-recipe	.5 cup	145	4.53	4.03	22.78	0	53	90	83		0.38	118
flaxseed	1 tbsp, whole	534	18.29	42.16	28.88	27.3	30	0	255	0	5.73	813
fondant, prepared-from-recipe	1 oz	373	0	0.02	93.18	0	11	0	3	0	0.01	4
frankfurter bf htd	1 hot dog	322	11.69	29.36	2.66	0	852	58	11	38	1.22	252
frankfurter meat	1 hot dog	290	10.26	25.76	4.17	0	1090	77	99		1.09	152
frankfurter meat htd	1 hot dog	278	9.77	24.31	4.9	0	1013	73	99		1.22	141
frankfurter, meat and poultry, cooked, boiled	1 hot dog	298	10.31	26.28	4.96	0	914	84	107	26	1.12	323

Food	Serving	Cals	Protein (g)	Fat (g)	Carbs (g)	Fiber (g)	Sodium (mg)	Cholesterol (mg)	Calcium (mg)	Vit D (IU)	Iron (mg)	Potassium (mg)
frankfurter, meat and poultry, cooked, grilled	1 hot dog	302	10.67	26.43	5.24	0	1079	85	118	27	1.15	387
french toast stks	3 pieces	340	6	17.74	41.21	1.4	400	0	53	0	1.92	111
french toast w/ butter	2 slices	264	7.66	13.9	26.7		380	86	54		1.4	131
french toast, frz, rth	1 oz	213	7.4	6.1	32.1	1.1	495	82	107		2.21	134
french toast, prep from recipe, made w/lofat (2%) milk	1 oz	229	7.7	10.8	25		479	116	100		1.67	134
fried chicken, breast, meat & skn & breading	1 breast, with skin	230	23.51	12.44	6.03	0.1	657	92	45	5	0.72	282
fried chicken, breast, meat only, skn & brding removed	1 breast, without skin	153	27.93	4.54	0	0	512	97	23	5	0.54	306
fried chicken, drmstk, meat only, skn & brding removed	1 drumstick, bone and skin removed	172	26.24	7.41	0	0	492	133	16	5	1.03	291
fried chicken, drumstk, meat & skn w/ breading	1 drumstick, with skin	267	21.13	16.92	7.59	0.5	591	111	24	5	0.99	253
fried chicken, skn & breading from all pieces	1 serving	398	14.11	29.22	19.56	0.3	965	82	92	7	1.12	230
fried chick, thigh, meat & skn & breading	1 thigh, with skin	274	19.23	18.07	8.68	0.1	747	106	54	7	1	240
fried chicken, thigh, meat only, skn & breding removed	1 thigh, without skin	178	23.21	9.41	0.24	0	577	125	24	8	0.91	248
fried chicken, wing, meat & skn & breading	1 wing, with skin	310	21.14	20.09	11.19	0.1	867	114	67	5	1.04	262
fried chicken, wing, meat only, skn & breading removed	1 wing, without skin	215	28.77	10.2	2.13	0	761	148	40	3	0.96	296
frijoles rojos volteados (refried bns, red, canned)	1 cup	144	5	6.93	15.47	4.7	375		33		1.95	310
frosted oat crl w/marshmallows	1 cup	400	7	3.33	84.7	4.3	533	0	333	143	15	207
frosting, glaz, chc, prep-frm-rcip, w/ butr, nfsmi recip no. c-32	2 tablespoon	359	1.42	7.17	72.18	1.1	132	18	32		0.6	130
frostings, choc, creamy, dry mix	1 package	389	1.3	5.2	92	2.4	76	0	11		1.19	180
frostings, choc, creamy, dry mix, prep w/ butter	2 tablespoon	408	1.11	13.06	71.8	1.9	124	24	12	7	0.93	143
frostings, choc, creamy, dry mix, prep w/ margarine	2 tablespoon	404	1.1	12.87	71.02	1.9	163	0	12		0.93	143
frostings, choc, creamy, rte	2 tbsp, creamy	397	1.1	17.6	63.2	0.9	183	0	8	0	1.42	196
frostings, coconut-nut, rte	.083 package	433	1.5	24	52.7	2.5	160	0	13	0	0.54	186
frostings, crm cheese-flavor, rte	2 tbsp, creamy	415	0.1	17.3	67.32	0	191	0	3		0.16	35
frostings, glaze, prepared-from-recipe	1 recipe, yield	341	0.44	0.53	83.65	0	6	1	17		0.03	30
frostings, vanilla, creamy, dry mix	1 package	410	0.3	4.9	93.8	0.1	13	0	3		0	7
frostings, vanilla, creamy, dry mix, prep w/ margarine	2 tablespoon	413	0.34	12.74	74.28	0.1	114	0	6		0.01	10
frostings, vanilla, creamy, rte	.083 package	418	0	16.23	67.89	0	184	0	3	0	0.16	34
frostings, white, fluffy, dry mix	1 package	371	2.3	0	94.9	0	234	0	4		0.09	117
frostings, white, fluffy, dry mix, prep w/h2o	1 package, yields	244	1.5	0	62.6	0	156	0	4		0.06	77
frozen yogurts, choc	1 cup	127	3	3.6	21.6	2.3	63	13	100	3	0.46	234
frozen yogurts, choc, soft-serve	.5 cup	160	4	6	24.9	2.2	98	5	147		1.25	261
frozen yogurts, flavors other than choc	1 cup	127	3	3.6	21.6	0	63	13	100	3	0.46	156
frozen yogurts, vanilla, soft-serve	.5 cup	159	4	5.6	24.2	0	87	2	143	4	0.3	211
fruit butters, apple	1 tbsp	173	0.39	0.3	42.47	1.5	15	0	14	0	0.31	91
fruit cocktail, cnd, ex hvy syrup, sol&liquids	.5 cup	88	0.39	0.07	22.89	1.1	6	0	6	0	0.28	86
fruit cocktail, cnd, ex lt syrup, sol&liquids	.5 cup	45	0.4	0.07	11.63	1.1	4	0	8	0	0.3	104
fruit flav drk containing , 3% fruit juc, w/ hi vit c	1 cup	27	0	0	6.67	0	36	0	3	0	0	31
fruit flav drk, less than 3% juc, not fort w/ vit c	1 cup	64	0	0	16.03	0	36	0	3	0	0	31
fruit flav drk, red sugar, > 3% fruit juc, hi vit c, add ca	1 cup	29	0	0.37	6.67	0	25	0	42	10	0	31

Food	Serving	Cals	Protein (g)	Fat (g)	Carbs (g)	Fiber (g)	Sodium (mg)	Cholesterol (mg)	Calcium (mg)	Vit D (IU)	Iron (mg)	Potassium (mg)
fruit juc drk, greater than 3% juc, hi vit c	1 cup	46	0.13	0.11	11.35	0.1	8	0	3	0	0.25	122
fruit juc drk, more 3% fruit juc, hi vit c & add thiamin	1 cup	54	0.13	0	13.16	0.1	61	0	3	0	0.25	122
fruit juc drk, red sugar, w/ vitamin e added	1 cup	39	0	0.07	10	0	2	0	5	0	0.04	11
fruit leather, pieces	1 oz	359	1	2.68	82.82	0	403	0	18	0	0.75	164
fruit leather, rolls	1 large	371	0.1	3	85.8	0	317	0	32	0	1.01	294
fruit punch drk, frz conc	1 fl oz	162	0.2	0	41.4	0.4	8	0	8		0.3	44
fruit punch drk, frz conc, prep w/ h2o	1 fl oz	46	0.06	0	11.66	0.1	5	0	4		0.09	13
fruit punch drk, w/ added nutr, cnd	1 fl oz	47	0	0	11.94	0.2	38	0	8	0	0.09	31
fruit punch drk, wo/ added nutr, cnd	6.75 fl oz	48	0	0	11.97	0	10	0	8	0	0.09	25
fruit punch juc drk, frz conc	1 fl oz	175	0.3	0.7	43.1	0.2	10	0	20		0.8	270
fruit punch juc drk, frz conc, prep w/ h2o	1 fl oz	42	0.07	0.17	11.4	0	5	0	7		0.2	66
fruit punch-flavor drk, pdr, wo/ added na, prep w/ h2o	1 fl oz	37	0	0.01	9.47	0	7	0	17		0.05	1
fruit snacks, w/ hi vit c	1 serving	352	0.08	0	87.97	0	23	0	0	0	0	8
fruit-flav drk, pdr, w/ hi vit c w/ other add vit, lo cal	1 tsp	227	0.25	0.16	91	2.2	14	0	800	0	0.08	2518
fruit-flavored drk, dry pdr mix, lo cal, w/ asprt	1 tsp	218	0.45	0.04	87.38	0.1	404	0	1047	0	0.08	498
fudge, choc marshmllw, prepared-from-recipe	1 piece	453	2.26	17.48	71.34	1.7	85	25	45		0.96	147
fudge, choc marshmllw, w/ prepared-by-recipe	1 oz	474	3.24	21.11	67.69	2.1	79	23	49		1.11	170
fudge, choc, prepared-from-recipe	1 piece	411	2.39	10.41	76.44	1.7	45	14	49	0	1.77	134
fudge, choc, w/ prepared-from-recipe	1 oz	461	4.38	18.93	67.93	2.5	39	12	57	0	1.97	183
fudge, pnut butter, prepared-from-recipe	1 piece	387	3.78	6.59	77.75	0.7	118	3	42		0.22	119
fudge, vanilla w/ nuts	1 oz	435	3	13.69	74.61	0.9	42	13	47	0	0.41	103
fudge, vanilla, prepared-from-recipe	1 oz	383	1.05	5.45	82.15	0	47	15	38	0	0.02	49
garlic bread, frz	1 slice, presliced	350	8.36	16.61	41.72	2.5	544	0	27	9	3.05	103
garlic powder	1 tsp	331	16.55	0.73	72.73	9	60	0	79	0	5.65	1193
garlic, raw	1 cup	149	6.36	0.5	33.06	2.1	17	0	181	0	1.7	401
gelatin dssrt, dry mix	3 oz	381	7.8	0	90.5	0	466	0	3	0	0.13	7
gelatin dssrt, dry mix, prep w/ h2o	.5 cup	62	1.22	0	14.19	0	75	0	3	0	0.02	1
gin, 90 proof	1 fl oz	263	0	0	0	0	2	0	0	0	0	0
ginger ale	1 fl oz	34	0	0	8.76	0	7	0	3	0	0.18	1
ginger root, raw	1 tsp	80	1.82	0.75	17.77	2	13	0	16	0	0.6	415
ginger, ground	1 tsp	335	8.98	4.24	71.62	14.1	27	0	114	0	19.8	1320
goji berries, dried	5 tbsp	349	14.26	0.39	77.06	13	298	0	190		6.8	
goose, domesticated, meat only, ckd, rstd	1 unit	238	28.97	12.67	0	0	76	96	14		2.87	388
goose, domesticated, meat&skn, ckd, rstd	1 cup, chopped or diced	305	25.16	21.92	0	0	70	91	13	3	2.83	329
granola bars, hard, plain	1 bar	471	10.1	19.8	64.4	5.3	294	0	61	0	2.95	336
granola bars, soft, uncoated, pln	1 bar	443	7.4	17.2	67.3	4.6	278	0	105		2.56	325
granola, homemade	1 cup	489	13.67	24.31	53.88	8.9	26	0	76	0	3.95	539
grape drk, cnd	1 fl oz	61	0	0	15.72	0	16	0	52	0	0.07	12
grape juc drk, cnd	1 fl oz	57	0	0	14.55	0.1	9	0	7	0	0.13	33
grape juc, cnd or btld, unswtnd, wo/ added vit c	1 cup	60	0.37	0.13	14.77	0.2	5	0	11	0	0.25	104
grape soda	1 fl oz	43	0	0	11.2	0	15	0	3		0.08	1
grapefruit juc, pink or red, w/ added ca	8 fl oz	38	0.5	0.1	8.69	0	1	0	146	0	0.2	162
grapefruit juc, white, raw	1 cup	39	0.5	0.1	9.2	0.1	1	0	9	0	0.2	162
grapefruit juice, pink, raw	1 cup	39	0.5	0.1	9.2		1	0	9	0	0.2	162
grapefruit, raw, pink&red, all areas	1 cup, sections with juice	42	0.77	0.14	10.66	1.6	0	0	22	0	0.08	135

Food	Serving	Cals	Protein (g)	Fat (g)	Carbs (g)	Fiber (g)	Sodium (mg)	Cholesterol (mg)	Calcium (mg)	Vit D (IU)	Iron (mg)	Potassium (mg)
grapefruit, raw, white, all areas	1 cup, sections with juice	33	0.69	0.1	8.41	1.1	0	0	12	0	0.06	148
grapes, muscadine, raw	1 grape	57	0.81	0.47	13.93	3.9	1		37		0.26	203
gravy, brown, dry	1 tbsp	367	10.74	9.61	59.38	2	4843	3	132		1.72	262
gravy, chicken, dry	1 tbsp	381	11.27	9.73	62.09		4152	19	146		1.33	404
griddle cake sndwch, egg, chs, & bacon	6.1 oz	272	12.03	13.19	26.19	0.8	718	147	109	13	1.65	158
griddle cake sndwch, egg, chs, & sausage	1 item	291	10.77	17.73	22.04	0.6	652	132	96	19	1.51	146
griddle cake sndwch, sausage	1 item	318	8.41	17.76	31.25	1	737	24	63	9	1.42	145
grilled chick filet sndwch, w/ lettuce, tomato & sprd	1 sandwich	182	17.34	4.57	16.78	0.9	427	40	62	2	1.58	197
grilled chick in tortilla, w/ lttc, chs, & ranch sau	1 wrap	222	13.77	10.31	18.43	0.9	577	41	93	2	1.45	192
grilled chick, bacon & tomo clb sndwch, w/ chs, lettuce, & mayo	1 sandwich	220	17.19	8.05	19.87	1.2	630	46	95	5	1.37	226
ground turkey, 85% ln, 15% fat, pan-broiled crumbles	3 oz	258	25.11	17.45	0	0	85	106	49	8	1.98	276
ground turkey, 85% ln, 15% fat, patties, brld	3 oz	249	25.88	16.2	0	0	81	105	48	8	2.04	242
ground turkey, 93% ln, 7% fat, pan-broiled crumbles	3 oz	213	27.1	11.6	0	0	90	104	31	8	1.56	304
ground turkey, 93% ln, 7% fat, patties, brld	3 oz	207	25.86	11.45	0	0	91	106	29	8	1.73	247
ground turkey, ckd	1 patty	203	27.37	10.4	0	0	78	93	28	8	1.52	294
ground turkey, fat free, pan-broiled crumbles	3 oz	151	31.69	2.71	0	0	61	71	6	8	1.02	357
ground turkey, fat free, patties, brld	1 patty	138	28.99	2.48	0	0	59	65	6	8	0.78	339
grouper, mxd sp, ckd, dry heat	3 oz	118	24.84	1.3	0	0	53	47	21		1.14	475
guavas, common, raw	1 cup	68	2.55	0.95	14.32	5.4	2	0	18	0	0.26	417
gumdrops, starch jelly pieces	1 cup, gumdrops	396	0	0	98.9	0.1	44	0	3	0	0.4	5
haddock, cooked, dry heat	1 fillet	90	19.99	0.55	0	0	261	66	14	23	0.21	351
haddock, smoked	1 oz, bone-less	116	25.23	0.96	0	0	763	77	49	34	1.4	415
halibut, atlantic&pacific, ckd, dry heat	3 oz	111	22.54	1.61	0	0	82	60	9	231	0.2	528
halibut, ckd, w/ skn (alaska native)	3 oz	113	22.13	2.73	0	0	86	75	33		0.36	501
halibut, greenland, ckd, dry heat	3 oz	239	18.42	17.74	0	0	103	59	4		0.85	344
ham and cheese spread	1 tbsp	245	16.18	18.53	2.28	0	1197	61	217		0.76	162
ham honey smoked ckd	1.94 oz	122	17.93	2.37	7.27	0	900	22	6		0.39	165
ham salad spread	1 tbsp	216	8.68	15.53	10.64	0	1075	37	8	26	0.59	150
ham, chopped, canned	1 oz	239	16.06	18.83	0.26	0	1280	49	7	24	0.95	284
ham, chopped, not canned	1 slice	180	16.5	10.3	4.2	0	1039	59	7	29	0.83	319
ham, minced	1 oz	263	16.28	20.68	1.84	0	1245	70	10	26	0.79	311
ham, sliced, pre-packaged, deli meat (96%fat free, h2o added)	1 slice	107	16.85	4.04	0.7	0	945	41	5	25	0.59	463
ham, sliced, reg (approx 11% fat)	56 grams	163	16.6	8.6	3.83	1.3	1143	57	24	29	1.02	287
ham, smoked, ex ln, lo na	1 slice	141	18.52	2.71	10.7	0	1062	50	5	27	0.76	330
hamburger, lrg, single patty, w/ condmnt	1 item	256	15.68	11.6	22.14	1.1	374	40	87	4	1.73	225
hamburger, lrg, triple patty, w/condmnt	1 sandwich	267	19.3	16.01	11.04		275	55	25		3.21	303
hamburger; double, lrg patty; w/ condmnt & veg	1 sandwich	239	15.17	11.75	17.82		350	54	45		2.59	252
hamburger; double, lrg paty; w/ condmnt, veg & mayo	1 item	252	13.94	15.66	13.74	1.4	289	46	35	4	2.8	192
hamburger; double, reg patty; w/ condmnt	1 item	268	14.8	15.1	18.02		345	48	43		2.58	245
hamburger; double, reg, patty; pln	1 item	295	17.08	14.36	24.1	0.9	414	47	102		2.88	226
hamburger; single, lrg patty; pln	1 sandwich	311	16.51	16.73	23.16		346	52	54		2.61	195
hamburger; single, lrg patty; w/ condmnt & veg	1 sandwich	235	11.85	12.55	18.35		378	40	44		2.26	220
hamburger; single, reg patty; pln	1 sandwich	297	16.52	12.01	31.5	1.7	331	33	62	2	3.06	197
hamburger; single, reg patty; w/ condmnt	1 sandwich	263	13.3	10.18	29.57	1.8	487	29	116	2	2.87	197

Food	Serving	Cals	Protein (g)	Fat (g)	Carbs (g)	Fiber (g)	Sodium (mg)	Cholesterol (mg)	Calcium (mg)	Vit D (IU)	Iron (mg)	Potassium (mg)
hamburger; single; reg patty; w/ condmnt & veg	1 item	254	11.74	12.25	24.81		458	24	57		2.39	206
hamburger; sng, reg ptty; dbl bn w/ cndmnt & spl sau	1 item	259	12.17	13.3	22.69	1.4	386	32	103		2.07	194
hazelnuts or filberts	1 cup, chopped	628	14.95	60.75	16.7	9.7	0	0	114	0	4.7	680
hemp sd, hulled	3 tbsp	553	31.56	48.75	8.67	4	5	0	70		7.95	1200
herring, atlantic, ckd, dry heat	1 fillet	203	23.03	11.59	0	0	115	77	74	214	1.41	419
herring, pacific, ckd, dry heat	1 fillet	250	21.01	17.79	0	0	95	99	106		1.44	542
herring, pacific, flsh, air-dried, pack oil (alaska native)	1 fillet	489	44.5	34.6	0							
hominy, canned, white	1 cup	72	1.48	0.88	14.26	2.5	345	0	10	0	0.62	9
hominy, canned, yellow	1 cup	72	1.48	0.88	14.26	2.5	345	0	10	0	0.62	9
honey	1 cup	304	0.3	0	82.4	0.2	4	0	6	0	0.42	52
honey-combed, w/ pnut butter	1 cup	486	8.72	28	67.41	1.9	174	0	21	0	0.71	220
horchata, as served in restaurant	1 cup	54	0.48	0.71	11.52	0	14		18		0.01	34
horchata, dry mix, unprep, var brands, all w/ morro seeds	1 tbsp	413	7.5	7.46	79.05	4	3	0	60	0	5.8	180
horseradish, prepared	1 tsp	48	1.18	0.69	11.29	3.3	420	0	56	0	0.42	246
hotdog, plain	1 sandwich	247	10.6	14.84	18.4		684	45	24		2.36	146
hotdog, w/chili	1 sandwich	260	11.85	11.79	27.45		421	45	17		2.88	146
hotdog, w/corn flr coating (corndog)	1 sandwich	263	9.6	10.8	31.88		556	45	58		3.53	150
hummus, commercial	1 tbsp	166	7.9	9.6	14.29	6	379	0	38	0	2.44	228
hummus, home prep	1 tablespoon	177	4.86	8.59	20.12	4	242	0	49	0	1.56	173
hush puppies	1 piece	296	6.16	13.25	40.21	2.9	813	0	100	0	2.55	256
hush puppies, prep from recipe	1 oz	337	7.7	13.5	46	2.8	668	45	278	0	3.04	144
ice creams, choc	3.5 fl oz	216	3.8	11	28.2	1.2	76	34	109	8	0.93	249
ice creams, french vanilla, soft-serve	4 fl oz	222	4.1	13	22.2	0.7	61	91	131	29	0.21	177
ice creams, strawberry	3.5 fl oz	192	3.2	8.4	27.6	0.9	60	29	120		0.21	188
ice creams, vanilla	1/2 cup	207	3.5	11	23.6	0.7	80	44	128	8	0.09	199
ice crm bar, choc or caramel covered, w/nuts	1 bar	323	4.4	20.2	30.9	0.6	92	1	252	7	0.72	238
ice crm bar, covered w/ choc & nuts	1 bar	303	5.62	25.84	11.89	1.1	56	56	90	9	1.21	304
ice crm bar, stk or nugget, w/ crunch coating	1 bar	358	2.11	25.26	37.12	1.1	84	16	63	3	0	71
ice crm cone, choc covered, w/ flavors other than choc	1 cone	354	5.21	21.88	34.38	1	94	21	63	3	0	222
ice crm cones, cake or wafer-type	1 oz	417	8.1	6.9	79	3	256	0	25	0	3.6	112
ice crm cones, sugar, rolled-type	1 oz	402	7.9	3.8	84.1	1.7	298	0	44	0	4.43	145
ice crm cookie sndwch	1 sandwich	240	3.7	7.4	39.6	1.2	162	6	73	0	1.1	68
ice crm sndwch	1 sandwich	237	4.29	8.57	37.14	0	129	21	86	0	0.26	115
ice crm sundae cone	1 cone	254	3	14	28.89	1	115	15	60	4	0.36	204
ice crm, bar or stk, choc covered	1 bar	331	4.1	24.1	24.5	0.8	68	28	119	7	0.29	305
ice crm, soft serve, choc	.5 cup	222	4.1	13	22.2	0.7	61	91	131	29	0.21	177
instant brkfst pdr, choc, not recon	1 tbsp	353	19.9	1.4	66.2	0.4	385	12	285	0	12.82	947
instant brkfst pdr, choc, sugar-free, not recon	1 tbsp	358	35.8	5.1	41	2	717	44	500	0	2.3	1705
jams & preserves, no sugar (with na saccharin), any flavor	1 cup	132	0.3	0.3	53.42	2.5	0	0	9	0	0.4	69
jams and preserves	1 tbsp	278	0.37	0.07	68.86	1.1	32	0	20	0	0.49	77
jellybeans	10 small	375	0	0.05	93.55	0.2	50	0	3	0	0.13	37
jerusalem-artichokes, raw	1 cup, slices	73	2	0.01	17.44	1.6	4	0	14	0	3.4	429
juice, appl & grape blend, w/ added vit c	8 fl oz	50	0.16	0.12	12.46	0.2	7	0	11	0	0.11	96
juice, appl, grape & pear blend, w/ added vit c & ca	8 fl oz	52	0.17	0.12	12.96	0.2	5	0	72	0	0.14	89
kale, ckd, bld, drnd, wo/salt	1 cup, chopped	28	1.9	0.4	5.63	2	23	0	72	0	0.9	228
kale, raw	1 cup, 1" pieces, loosely packed	49	4.28	0.93	8.75	3.6	38	0	150	0	1.47	491
ketchup	1 tbsp	101	1.04	0.1	27.4	0.3	907	0	15	0	0.35	281
kielbasa, fully ckd, grilled	3 oz	337	12.45	29.68	5.03	0	1062	73	42	35	0.99	306

Food	Serving	Cals	Protein (g)	Fat (g)	Carbs (g)	Fiber (g)	Sodium (mg)	Cholesterol (mg)	Calcium (mg)	Vit D (IU)	Iron (mg)	Potassium (mg)
kielbasa, fully ckd, pan-fried	1 link	333	12.36	29.43	4.78	0	1046	73	40	9	0.93	304
kiwi strawberry juc drk	16 fl oz	47	0	0	12.26	0	11	0	0	0	0.15	14
kiwifruit, grn, raw	1 cup, sliced	61	1.14	0.52	14.66	3	3	0	34	0	0.31	312
kumquats, raw	1 fruit, without refuse	71	1.88	0.86	15.9	6.5	10	0	62	0	0.86	186
lamb, aus, frsh, leg, hindshank, heel on, bne-in, ln & ft, 1/8", brsd	3 oz	204	29.52	9.5	0	0	84	110	6	0	2	192
lamb, aus, frsh, leg, hindshank, heel on, bone-in, ln, 1/8", brsd	3 oz	174	30.73	5.63	0	0	86	111	5	0	2.02	192
lamb, aus, frsh, leg, trotter off, bone-in, ln & fat, 1/8" fat, rstd	3 oz	226	30.15	11.64	0.08	0	77	113	4	0	2.41	291
lamb, aus, frsh, leg, trotter off, bone-in, ln, 1/8" fat, ckd, rstd	3 oz	215	32.08	9.59	0	0	80	117	4	0	2.55	308
lamb, aus, frsh, rack, rst, frenched, bne-in, ln & ft, 1/8", rstd	3 oz	291	25.96	20.77	0	0	65	97	7	0	2.47	228
lamb, aus, frsh, rack, rst, frenched, bone-in, ln, 1/8" fat, ckd, rstd	3 oz	244	28.01	14.64	0	0	67	96	6	0	2.63	237
lamb, aus, frsh, rack, rst, frnched, dnuded, bne-in, ln & ft, 0", rstd	3 oz	193	25.95	9.91	0	0	71	97	7	0	1.92	227
lamb, aus, frsh, rack, rst, frnched, dnuded, bone-in, ln, 0", ckd, rstd	3 oz	175	26.52	7.63	0	0	72	97	7	0	1.94	230
lamb, aus, frsh, rib chop, frenched, bne-in, ln & fat, 1/8", grilled	3 oz	305	28.48	21.2	0	0	79	91	11	0	2.24	292
lamb, aus, frsh, rib chop, frnched, bone-in, ln, 1/8", ckd, grilled	3 oz	234	32.16	11.68	0	0	85	92	11	0	2.36	320
lamb, aus, frsh, rib chop, frnched, dnuded, bone-in, ln, 0", grilled	3 oz	236	33.17	11.5	0	0	85	103	10	0	2.46	294
lamb, aus, imp, frsh, comp of rtl cuts, ln, 1/8"fat, ckd	3 oz	201	26.71	9.63	0		80	87	16		2.05	318
lamb, aus, imp, frsh, comp of rtl cuts, ln&fat, 1/8"fat, ckd	3 oz	256	24.52	16.82	0		76	87	17		1.93	301
lambsquarters, ckd, bld, drnd, wo/salt	1 cup, chopped	32	3.2	0.7	5	2.1	29	0	258	0	0.7	288
lard	1 tbsp	902	0	100	0	0	0	95	0	102	0	0
lasagna w/ meat & sau, frz entree	1 piece, side	124	6.63	4.42	14.39	1.4	347	14	73	1	0.65	184
lasagna w/ meat sau, frz, prep	1 piece, side	135	7.28	4.92	15.36	1.7	373	17	88	1	0.71	196
leavening agents, baking pdr, double-acting, na al sulfate	1 tsp	53	0	0	27.7	0.2	10600	0	5876	0	11.02	20
leavening agents, baking soda	1 tsp	0	0	0	0	0	27360	0	0	0	0	0
leavening agents, yeast, baker's, active dry	1 tsp	325	40.44	7.61	41.22	26.9	51	0	30	0	2.17	955
leeks, (bulb&lower leaf-portion), ckd, bld, drnd, wo/salt	1 leek	31	0.81	0.2	7.62	1	10	0	30	0	1.1	87
leeks, (bulb&lower leaf-portion), raw	1 cup	61	1.5	0.3	14.15	1.8	20	0	59	0	2.1	180
lemon juc from conc, btld, concord	1 tbsp	24	0.4	0.07	5.37		29		8		0.06	112
lemon juc from conc, btld, real lemon	1 tbsp	17	0.47	0.07	5.66	0.7	26		9		0.06	109
lemon juc from conc, cnd or btld	1 tbsp	17	0.45	0.07	5.62	0.7	24	0	10	0	0.06	109
lemon juice, raw	1 cup	22	0.35	0.24	6.9	0.3	1	0	6	0	0.08	103
lemon peel, raw	1 tbsp	47	1.5	0.3	16	10.6	6	0	134	0	0.8	160
lemon-lime soda, no caffeine	1 fl oz	41	0.09	0	10.42	0	10	0	2	0	0.02	1
lemonade fruit juc drk lt, fort w/ vit e & c	8 fl oz	21	0	0	5	0	5	0	2	0	0	10
lemonade-flavor drk, pdr	1 serving	380	0	1.01	97.9	0	130	0	11	0	0.17	39
lemonade-flavor drk, pdr, prep w/ h2o	1 fl oz	27	0	0.07	6.9	0	13	0	4	0	0.01	3
lemonade, frz conc, pink	1 fl oz	192	0.22	0.69	48.86	0.3	4	0	8	0	0.08	76
lemonade, frz conc, pink, prep w/h2o	1 fl oz	43	0.05	0.15	10.81	0.1	4	0	4	0	0.02	17
lemonade, frz conc, white	1 fl oz	196	0.22	0.7	49.89	0.3	7	0	7	0	0.09	72
lemonade, frz conc, white, prep w/h2o	1 fl oz	40	0.07	0.04	10.42	0	4	0	4		0.16	15
lemonade, pdr	1 serving	376	0	1.05	97.57	0.4	51	0	20	0	0.19	147
lemonade, pdr, prep w/h2o	1 fl oz	14	0	0.04	3.59	0	6	0	4	0	0.01	6
lemons, raw, without peel	1 cup, sections	29	1.1	0.3	9.32	2.8	2	0	26	0	0.6	138
lentils, mature ckd, bld, wo/salt	1 cup	116	9.02	0.38	20.13	7.9	2	0	19	0	3.33	369

Food	Serving	Cals	Protein (g)	Fat (g)	Carbs (g)	Fiber (g)	Sodium (mg)	Cholesterol (mg)	Calcium (mg)	Vit D (IU)	Iron (mg)	Potassium (mg)
lentils, sprouted, ckd, stir-fried, wo/salt	1 cup	101	8.8	0.45	21.25		10	0	14	0	3.1	284
lettuce, butterhead (incl boston&bibb types), raw	1 cup, shredded or chopped	13	1.35	0.22	2.23	1.1	5	0	35	0	1.24	238
lettuce, cos or romaine, raw	1 cup, shredded	17	1.23	0.3	3.29	2.1	8	0	33	0	0.97	247
lettuce, grn leaf, raw	1 cup, shredded	15	1.36	0.15	2.87	1.3	28	0	36	0	0.86	194
lettuce, iceberg (incl crisphead types), raw	1 cup, shredded	14	0.9	0.14	2.97	1.2	10	0	18	0	0.41	141
lettuce, red leaf, raw	1 cup, shredded	16	1.33	0.22	2.26	0.9	25	0	33	0	1.2	187
lima bns, immat ckd, bld, drnd, wo/salt	1 cup	123	6.81	0.32	23.64	5.4	17	0	32	0	2.45	570
lime juc, cnd or btld, unswtnd	1 cup	21	0.25	0.23	6.69	0.4	16	0	12	0	0.23	75
lime juice, raw	1 cup	25	0.42	0.07	8.42	0.4	2	0	14	0	0.09	117
limeade, frz conc, prep w/h2o	1 fl oz	52	0	0	13.79	0	3	0	2		0	10
limeade, hi caffeine	1 cup	18	0	0.11	4.16	0	40	0	2	0	0.03	19
limes, raw	1 lime	30	0.7	0.2	10.54	2.8	2	0	33	0	0.6	102
lo cal, cola or pepper-type, w/ asprt, caffeine, lo cal	1 fl oz	2	0.11	0.03	0.29	0	8	0	3	0	0.11	8
lo cal, other than cola or pepper, w/ asprt, caffeine, lo cal	1 fl oz	0	0.1	0	0	0	6	0	4	0	0.04	2
lobster, northern, ckd, moist heat	1 cup	89	19	0.86	0	0	486	146	96	1	0.29	230
luncheon meat, pork, canned	1 oz	334	12.5	30.3	2.1	0	1289	62	6	22	0.72	215
luncheon sausage, pork&bf	1 slice	260	15.38	20.9	1.58	0	1182	64	13		1.43	245
mac & chs, dry mix, prep w/ 2% milk & 80% stk margarine dry mx	1 cup	190	4.89	8.28	23.93	1.2	338	3	63		0.99	129
macadamia dry rstd, w/salt	1 cup, whole or halves	716	7.79	76.08	12.83	8	353	0	70	0	2.65	363
macadamia dry rstd, wo/salt	1 cup, whole or halves	718	7.79	76.08	13.38	8	4	0	70	0	2.65	363
macadamia raw	1 cup, whole or halves	718	7.91	75.77	13.82	8.6	5	0	85	0	3.69	368
macaroni & chs dinner w/ dry sau mix, boxed, unckd	1 cup	379	13.86	4.82	70.12	3.2	680	7	146	0	2.75	347
macaroni & chs, box mix w/ chs sau, prep	1 cup, prepared	164	6.68	4.99	23.1	1.2	460	8	85		1.17	80
macaroni & chs, cnd entree	7.5 oz	82	3.38	2.46	11.52	0.5	302	6	35	0	0.9	84
macaroni & chs, cnd, microwavable	7.5 oz	134	5.98	5.99	13.96	0.4	335	20	57		0.91	72
macaroni & chs, frz entree	1 cup	149	5.6	6.41	17.28	1.1	290	10	114	0	0.57	95
mackerel, atlantic, ckd, dry heat	1 fillet	262	23.85	17.81	0	0	83	75	15		1.57	401
mackerel, jack, cnd, drnd sol	1 oz, bone-less	156	23.19	6.3	0	0	379	79	241	292	2.04	194
mackerel, king, ckd, dry heat	3 oz	134	26	2.56	0	0	203	68	40		2.28	558
mackerel, pacific&jack, mxd sp, ckd, dry heat	1 oz, bone-less	201	25.73	10.12	0	0	110	60	29	457	1.49	521
mahimahi, ckd, dry heat	3 oz	109	23.72	0.9	0	0	113	94	19		1.45	533
malt bev, incl non-alcoholic beer	1 fl oz	37	0.21	0.12	8.05	0	13	0	7	0	0.06	8
malt drk mix, choc, w/ added nutr, pdr, prep w/ whl milk	1 cup	87	3.29	3.26	11.19	0.4	87	10	139	123	1.42	217
malt liquor bev	1 bottle	40	0.35	0	0	0	3	0	3	0	0.03	33
malted drk mix, choc, pdr	3 tsp	411	5.1	4.76	86.94	4.8	190	1	60	0	2.28	618
malted drk mix, choc, pdr, prep w/ whl milk	1 cup	85	3.37	3.29	11.2	0.5	60	10	98		0.21	172
malted drk mix, nat, pdr, dairy based.	3 tsp	428	14.29	9.52	71.21	0.1	405	24	298	0	0.7	758
malted drk mix, nat, pdr, prep w/ whl milk	1 cup	88	3.86	3.62	10.23	0.1	79	12	117		0.09	183
malted drk mix, nat, w/ add nutr, pdr, prep w/ whl milk	1 cup	86	3.67	3.21	10.67	0	72	11	123		1.36	200
mangos, raw	1 cup, pieces	60	0.82	0.38	14.98	1.6	1	0	11	0	0.16	168
maraschino cherries, cnd, drnd	1 cherry	165	0.22	0.21	41.97	3.2	4	0	54	0	0.43	21
margarine-like, margarine-butter blend, soybn oil & butter	1 tbsp	727	0.31	80.32	0.77	0	719	12	10	1	0.04	22

Food	Serving	Cals	Protein (g)	Fat (g)	Carbs (g)	Fiber (g)	Sodium (mg)	Cholesterol (mg)	Calcium (mg)	Vit D (IU)	Iron (mg)	Potassium (mg)
margarine-like, veg oil sprd, stk or tub, swtnd	1 tablespoon	534	0	52	16.7	0	542	0	0	0	0	30
margarine, reg, 80% fat, comp, stk, w/ salt	1 tbsp	717	0.16	80.71	0.7	0	751	0	3	0	0.06	18
margarine, reg, 80% fat, comp, stk, w/ salt, w/ added vitamin d	1 tablespoon	717	0.16	80.71	0.7	0	751	0	3	429	0.06	18
margarine, reg, 80% fat, comp, stk, wo/ salt	1 tbsp	717	0.16	80.71	0.7	0	2	0	3	0	0.06	18
margarine, reg, 80% fat, comp, stk, wo/ salt, w/ added vitamin d	1 tbsp	717	0.16	80.71	0.7	0	2	0	3	429	0.06	18
margarine, reg, 80% fat, comp, tub, w/ salt	1 tbsp	713	0.22	80.17	0.75	0	657	0	3	0	0	17
margarine, reg, 80% fat, comp, tub, w/ salt, w/ added vitamin d	1 tbsp	713	0.22	80.17	0.75	0	657	0	3	429	0	17
margarine, reg, 80% fat, comp, tub, wo/ salt	1 tbsp	713	0.22	80.17	0.75	0	28	0	3	0	0	17
margarine, reg, hard, soybn (hydr)	1 tsp	719	0.9	80.5	0.9	0	943	0	30		0	42
marshmallows	1 cup, of miniature	318	1.8	0.2	81.3	0.1	80	0	3	0	0.23	5
mayonnaise drsng, no chol	1 tbsp	688	0	77.8	0.3	0	486	0	7	0	0.23	14
mayonnaise, lo na, lo cal or diet	1 tbsp	231	0.3	19.2	16	0	110	24	0	0	0	10
mayonnaise, made with tofu	1 tbsp	322	5.95	31.79	3.06	1.1	773	0	53	0	0.27	66
meal supp drk, cnd, pnut flavor	1 cup	101	3.5	3.07	14.74		54		110		2.2	160
meatballs, frz, italian style	3 oz	286	14.4	22.21	8.06	2.3	666	66	80	2	1.77	296
melons, cantaloupe, raw	1 cup, balls	34	0.84	0.19	8.16	0.9	16	0	9	0	0.21	267
melons, honeydew, raw	1 cup	36	0.54	0.14	9.09	0.8	18	0	6	0	0.17	228
milk bev, red fat, flav & swtnd, rtd, added ca, vit a & d	1 cup	77	3.05	1.83	12.08	0.4	49	8	164	45	0.03	130
milk choc	1 bar, miniature	535	7.65	29.66	59.4	3.4	79	23	189	0	2.35	372
milk choc coatd coffee bns	1 oz	549	7.41	33.18	55.25	5.7	70	20	169	0	2.29	413
milk choc coatd pnuts	1 cup	519	13.1	33.5	49.7	4.7	41	9	104	0	1.31	502
milk choc coatd raisins	1 cup	390	4.1	14.8	68.4	3.1	36	3	86	0	1.71	514
milk choc, w/almonds	1 bar, (1.45 oz)	526	9	34.4	53.4	6.2	74	19	224	0	1.63	444
milk choc, w/rice crl	1 bar, (1.4 oz)	511	7.64	29.37	59.67	3.3	86	23	187	0	2.65	370
milk shakes, thick choc	1 fl oz	119	3.05	2.7	21.15	0.3	111	11	132	41	0.31	224
milk shakes, thick vanilla	1 fl oz	112	3.86	3.03	17.75	0	95	12	146	48	0.1	183
milk, bttrmlk, fluid, whl	1 cup	62	3.21	3.31	4.88	0	105	11	115	52	0.03	135
milk, choc bev, hot cocoa, homemade	1 cup	77	3.52	2.34	10.74	1	44	8	114	45	0.42	197
milk, cnd, cond, swtnd	1 fl oz	321	7.91	8.7	54.4	0	127	34	284	6	0.19	371
milk, cnd, evap, nonfat, w/ added vit a & vitamin d	1 fl oz	78	7.55	0.2	11.35	0	115	4	290	79	0.29	332
milk, dry, whl, w/ added vitamin d	.25 cup	496	26.32	26.71	38.42	0	371	97	912	420	0.47	1330
milk, fluid, 1% fat, wo/ added vit a & vit d	1 cup	42	3.37	0.97	4.99	0	44	5	125	1	0.03	150
milk, fluid, nonfat, ca fort (fat free or skim)	1 cup	35	3.4	0.18	4.85	0	52	2	204	47	0.04	166
milk, goat, fluid, w/ added vitamin d	1 fl oz	69	3.56	4.14	4.45	0	50	11	134	51	0.05	204
milk, imitation, non-soy	1 cup	46	1.6	2	5.3	0	55	0	82	42	0.1	150
milk, nonfat, fluid, w/ added vit a & vit d (fat free or skim)	1 cup	34	3.37	0.08	4.96	0	42	2	122	47	0.03	156
milk, red fat, fluid, 2% milkfat, prot fort, w/ added vit a & d	1 cup	56	3.95	1.98	5.49	0	59	8	143	40	0.06	182
milkshake mix, dry, not choc	1 tbsp	329	23.5	2.6	52.9	1.6	780	14	880	0	7.7	2200
miso	1 tbsp	198	12.79	6.01	25.37	5.4	3728	0	57	0	2.49	210
mixed nuts dry rstd, w/ psalt added, chosen roaster	1 cup	632	18	58.8	19.02	7.1	113		106		3.22	585
mixed nuts, dry rstd, w/pw/salt	1 cup	594	17.3	51.45	25.35	9	345	0	70	0	3.7	693
mixed nuts, dry rstd, w/pwo/salt	1 cup	607	19.5	53.5	22.42	6.4	4	0	87	0	3.73	643
mixed nuts, oil rstd, w/pw/salt	1 cup	607	20.04	53.95	21.05	7	5	0	117	0	2.61	632
mixed nuts, oil rstd, wo/pwo/salt	1 cup	615	15.52	56.17	22.27	5.5	11	0	106	0	2.57	544
molasses	1 cup	290	0	0.1	74.73	0	37	0	205	0	4.72	1464
monkcooked, dry heat	3 oz	97	18.56	1.95	0	0	23	32	10		0.41	513

214

Food	Serving	Cals	Protein (g)	Fat (g)	Carbs (g)	Fiber (g)	Sodium (mg)	Cholesterol (mg)	Calcium (mg)	Vit D (IU)	Iron (mg)	Potassium (mg)
mousse, choc, prepared-from-recipe	1 recipe, yield	225	4.14	16	16.07	0.6	38	140	96		0.55	143
muffin, blueberry, commly prep, low-fat	1 muffin, small	255	4.23	4.22	50.05	4.2	413	28	35	3	2	96
muffins, blueberry, commly prep (includes mini-muffins)	1 oz	375	4.49	16.07	53	1.1	336	30	44	4	1.3	121
muffins, blueberry, prep from recipe, made w/lofat (2%) milk	1 oz	285	6.5	10.8	40.7		441	37	189		2.27	123
muffins, corn, commly prep	1 oz	305	5.9	8.4	51	3.4	467	26	74	0	2.81	69
muffins, corn, dry mix, prep	1 oz	321	7.4	10.2	49.1	2.4	795	62	75		1.94	131
muffins, corn, prep from recipe, made w/lofat (2%) milk	1 oz	316	7.1	12.3	44.2		585	42	259		2.61	145
muffins, oat bran	1 oz	270	7	7.4	48.3	4.6	393	0	63	0	4.2	507
muffins, pln, prep from recipe, made w/lofat (2%) milk	1 oz	296	6.9	11.4	41.4	2.7	467	39	200		2.39	121
muffins, wheat bran, toaster-type w/ raisins, tstd	1 oz	313	5.5	9.4	55.5	8.2	527	9	39		2.83	177
mullet, striped, ckd, dry heat	1 fillet	150	24.81	4.86	0	0	71	63	31		1.41	458
mushrooms, chanterelle, raw	1 cup	38	1.49	0.53	6.86	3.8	9		15	212	3.47	506
mushrooms, portabella, grilled	1 cup, sliced	29	3.28	0.58	4.44	2.2	11	0	3	14	0.4	437
mushrooms, portabella, raw	1 cup, diced	22	2.11	0.35	3.87	1.3	9	0	3	10	0.31	364
mushrooms, shiitake, ckd, w/salt	1 cup, pieces	56	1.56	0.22	14.39	2.1	240	0	3	28	0.44	117
mushrooms, shiitake, ckd, wo/salt	1 cup, pieces	56	1.56	0.22	14.39	2.1	4	0	3	28	0.44	117
mushrooms, shiitake, raw	1 piece, whole	34	2.24	0.49	6.79	2.5	9		2	18	0.41	304
mushrooms, shiitake, stir-fried	1 cup, whole	39	3.45	0.35	7.68	3.6	5	0	2	21	0.53	326
mushrooms, white, ckd, bld, drnd, w/ salt	1 cup, pieces	28	2.17	0.47	5.29	2.2	238	0	6	8	1.74	356
mushrooms, white, ckd, bld, drnd, wo/ salt	1 cup, pieces	28	2.17	0.47	5.29	2.2	2	0	6	8	1.74	356
mushrooms, white, raw	1 cup, pieces or slices	22	3.09	0.34	3.26	1	5	0	3	7	0.5	318
mushrooms, white, stir-fried	1 cup, sliced	26	3.58	0.33	4.04	1.8	12	0	4	8	0.25	396
mussel, blue, ckd, moist heat	3 oz	172	23.8	4.48	7.39	0	369	56	33		6.72	268
mustard grns, ckd, bld, drnd, wo/salt	1 cup, chopped	26	2.56	0.47	4.51	2	9	0	118	0	0.87	162
nachos, w/ chs, bns, ground bf, & tomatoes	1 serving	219	6.21	12.48	21.39	3.7	348	14	47	2	1.01	298
nachos, w/chs	1 serving	343	4.32	21.5	34.91	3.2	313	3	63	0	0.75	362
nectarines, raw	1 cup, slices	44	1.06	0.32	10.55	1.7	0	0	6	0	0.28	201
noodles, chinese, cellophane or long rice (mung bns), dehyd	1 cup	351	0.16	0.06	86.09	0.5	10	0	25	0	2.17	10
noodles, chinese, chow mein	.5 cup, dry	475	8.11	15.43	72.8	3.7	1174	0	20	0	4.73	120
noodles, egg, ckd, enr, w/ salt	1 cup	138	4.54	2.07	25.16	1.2	165	29	12		1.47	38
noodles, egg, ckd, unenr, w/ salt	1 cup	138	4.54	2.07	25.16	1.2	165	29	12		0.6	38
noodles, japanese, soba, ckd	1 cup	99	5.06	0.1	21.44		60	0	4	0	0.48	35
nougat, w/ almonds	1 piece	398	3.33	1.67	92.39	3.3	33	0	32	0	0.59	105
nutmeg, ground	1 tsp	525	5.84	36.31	49.29	20.8	16	0	184	0	3.04	350
nutritional shake mix, hi prot, pdr	1 tbsp	392	53.57	10.71	20.38	0	1214	0	714	500	22.5	1000
oat bran, cooked	1 cup	40	3.21	0.86	11.44	2.6	1	0	10	0	0.88	92
oat flr, part debranned	1 cup	404	14.66	9.12	65.7	6.5	19	0	55	0	4	371
oats	1 cup	389	16.89	6.9	66.27	10.6	2	0	54	0	4.72	429
oats, inst, fort, pln, prep w/ h2o	1 cup, cooked	68	2.37	1.36	11.67	1.7	49	0	80	0	5.96	61
oats, inst, fort, w/ cinn & spice, dry	1 packet	369	9.53	4.84	76.08	8	434	0	234	0	8.46	284
oats, inst, fort, w/ cinn & spice, prep w/h2o	1 cup	96	2.37	1.21	18.95	2	111	0	61	0	2.11	71
oats, inst, fort, w/ raisins & spice, dry	1 packet	360	8.45	4.03	76.33	5.7	462	0	228	0	9.43	362
oats, inst, fort, w/ raisins & spice, prep w/h2o	1 cup	88	1.98	0.95	17.91	1.3	111	0	56	0	2.21	85
oats, reg & quick & inst, unenr, ckd w/ h2o, w/ salt	1 cup	71	2.54	1.52	12	1.7	71	0	9		0.9	70
oats, reg & quick, not fort, dry	1 cup	379	13.15	6.52	67.7	10.1	6	0	52	0	4.25	362
oats, reg & quick, unenr, ckd w/ h2o, wo/ salt	1 cup	71	2.54	1.52	12	1.7	4	0	9	0	0.9	70
ocean perch, atlantic, ckd, dry heat	1 fillet	96	18.51	1.87	0	0	347	63	34	58	0.27	226

Food	Serving	Cals	Protein (g)	Fat (g)	Carbs (g)	Fiber (g)	Sodium (mg)	Cholesterol (mg)	Calcium (mg)	Vit D (IU)	Iron (mg)	Potassium (mg)
octopus, common, ckd, moist heat	3 oz	164	29.82	2.08	4.4	0	460	96	106	0	9.54	630
oil, almond	1 tablespoon	884	0	100	0	0	0	0	0	0	0	0
oil, avocado	1 tbsp	884	0	100	0	0	0		0		0	0
oil, canola	1 tbsp	884	0	100	0	0	0	0	0	0	0	0
oil, cocnt	1 tbsp	892	0	99.06	0	0	0	0	1	0	0.05	0
oil, cocoa butter	1 tablespoon	884	0	100	0	0	0	0	0		0	0
oil, cooking & salad, enova, 80% diglycerides	1 tbsp	884	0	100	0		0					
oil, corn and canola	1 tbsp	884	0	100	0	0	0	0	0	0	0	0
oil, corn, industrial & rtl, allpurp salad or cooking	1 tbsp	900	0	100	0	0	0	0	0	0	0	0
oil, corn, peanut, and olive	1 tablespoon	884	0	100	0	0	0	0	0	0	0.13	0
oil, cttnsd, salad or cooking	1 tablespoon	884	0	100	0	0	0	0	0	0	0	0
oil, cupu assu	1 tablespoon	884	0	100	0	0	0	0	0			0
oil, flaxseed, cold pressed	1 tbsp	884	0.11	99.98	0	0	0	0	1	0	0	0
oil, flaxseed, contains added sliced flaxseed	1 tablespoon	878	0.37	99.01	0.39		6	0	9		0.34	31
oil, grapeseed	1 tablespoon	884	0	100	0	0	0	0	0		0	0
oil, hazelnut	1 tablespoon	884	0	100	0	0	0	0	0		0	0
oil, olive, salad or cooking	1 tablespoon	884	0	100	0	0	2	0	1	0	0.56	1
oil, palm	1 tbsp	884	0	100	0	0	0	0	0		0.01	0
oil, sesame, salad or cooking	1 tablespoon	884	0	100	0	0	0	0	0	0	0	0
oil, soybn, salad or cooking	1 tbsp	884	0	100	0	0	0	0	0	0	0.05	0
oil, soybn, salad or cooking, (partially hydrogenated)	1 tbsp	884	0	100	0	0	0	0	0	0	0	0
okra, ckd, bld, drnd, wo/salt	.5 cup, slices	22	1.87	0.21	4.51	2.5	6	0	77	0	0.28	135
okra, frz, ckd, bld, drnd, wo/salt	.5 cup, slices	29	1.63	0.24	6.41	2.1	3	0	74	0	0.52	184
okra, raw	1 cup	33	1.93	0.19	7.45	3.2	7	0	82	0	0.62	299
onion powder	1 tsp	341	10.41	1.04	79.12	15.2	73	0	384	0	3.9	985
onion rings, breaded, par fr, frz, prep, htd in oven	1 cup	276	4.14	14.3	33.79	2.2	370	0	31	0	1.25	123
onion rings, breaded&fried	18 onion rings	411	3.86	25.23	43.58	2.7	776	0	115	0	0.78	167
onions, ckd, bld, drnd, wo/salt	1 cup	44	1.36	0.19	10.15	1.4	3	0	22	0	0.24	166
onions, dehydrated flakes	1 tbsp	349	8.95	0.46	83.28	9.2	21	0	257	0	1.55	1622
onions, raw	1 cup, chopped	40	1.1	0.1	9.34	1.7	4	0	23	0	0.21	146
orange & apricot juc drk, cnd	1 fl oz	51	0.3	0.1	12.7	0.1	2	0	5	0	0.1	80
orange brkfst drk, rtd, w/ added nutr	1 fl oz	53	0	0	13.2	0.1	54	0	100	0	0.05	83
orange drk, brkfst type, w/ juc & pulp, frz conc	1 fl oz	153	0.4	0	39	0.1	26	0	399	0	0.26	465
orange drk, brkfst type, w/ juc & pulp, frz conc, pre w/ h2o	1 fl oz	45	0.12	0	11.32	0	10	0	118		0.08	167
orange drk, cnd, w/ added vit c	1 fl oz	49	0	0.07	12.34	0	3	0	5	0	0.04	18
orange juc drk	1 cup	54	0.2	0	13.41	0.2	2	0	2		0.11	42
orange juc, chilled, incl from conc	1 cup	49	0.68	0.12	11.54	0.3	2	0	11	0	0.13	178
orange juc, cnd, unswtnd	1 cup	47	0.68	0.15	11.01	0.3	4	0	10	0	0.1	184
orange juc, lt, no pulp	8 fl oz	21	0.21	0	5.42	0	4	0	0	0	0	188
orange juice, raw	1 cup	45	0.7	0.2	10.4	0.2	1	0	11	0	0.2	200
orange-flav drk, brkfst type, w/ pulp, frz conc, pre w/ h2o	1 fl oz	49	0.03	0.14	12.21	0	10	0	39		0.08	124
orange-flavo drk, brkfst type, w/ pulp, frz con. not manuf.	1 fl oz	172	0.1	0.5	42.9	0.2	24	0	130	0	0.26	435
orange-flavor drk, brkfst type, lo cal, pdr	8 fl oz prepared	217	3.6	0	85.9	3.8	81	0	1378		0.07	3132
orange-flavor drk, brkfst type, pdr	2 tbsp	386	0	0	98.94	0.4	17	0	385	0	0.02	190
orange-flavor drk, brkfst type, pdr, prep w/h2o	1 fl oz	49	0	0	12.65	0.1	5	0	52		0	25
oranges, raw, all comm var	1 cup	47	0.94	0.12	11.75	2.4	0	0	40	0	0.1	181
oven-roasted chick breast roll	2 oz	134	14.59	7.65	1.79	0	883	39	6		0.32	324
oyster, eastern, canned	3 oz	68	7.06	2.47	3.91	0	112	55	45	1	6.7	229
oyster, eastern, ckd, breaded&fried	3 oz	199	8.77	12.58	11.62		417	71	62		6.95	244
oyster, eastern, farmed, ckd, dry heat	3 oz	79	7	2.12	7.28	0	163	38	56		7.77	152
oyster, eastern, wild, ckd, moist heat	3 oz	102	11.42	3.42	5.45	0	166	79	116	2	9.21	139

Food	Serving	Cals	Protein (g)	Fat (g)	Carbs (g)	Fiber (g)	Sodium (mg)	Cholesterol (mg)	Calcium (mg)	Vit D (IU)	Iron (mg)	Potassium (mg)
oyster, pacific, raw	1 medium	81	9.45	2.3	4.95	0	106	50	8		5.11	168
pancakes pln, frz, rth (includes buttermilk)	1 oz	233	5.23	6.83	37.75	1	461	18	78	0	5.67	90
pancakes, blueberry, prep from recipe	1 oz	222	6.1	9.2	29		412	56	206		1.72	138
pancakes, bttrmlk, prep from recipe	1 oz	227	6.8	9.3	28.7		522	58	157		1.7	145
pancakes, pln, dry mix, complete (incl bttrmlk)	.333 cup	368	9.77	3.1	73.65	2.9	1082	2	344		3.6	191
pancakes, pln, dry mix, complete, prep	1 oz	194	5.2	2.5	36.7	1.3	628	12	126		1.56	175
papayas, raw	1 cup	43	0.47	0.26	10.82	1.7	8	0	20	0	0.25	182
paprika	1 tsp	282	14.14	12.89	53.99	34.9	68	0	229	0	21.14	2280
parsley, dried	1 tsp	292	26.63	5.48	50.64	26.7	452	0	1140	0	22.04	2683
parsley, frsh	1 cup, chopped	36	2.97	0.79	6.33	3.3	56	0	138	0	6.2	554
parsnips, ckd, bld, drnd, wo/salt	.5 cup, slices	71	1.32	0.3	17.01	3.6	10	0	37	0	0.58	367
parsnips, raw	1 cup, slices	75	1.2	0.3	17.99	4.9	10	0	36	0	0.59	375
pasta mix, classic bf, unprep	1 cup	354	12.32	1.78	72.2	2	1537	0	21	0	2.71	342
pasta mix, classic cheeseburger macaroni, unprep	1 cup	349	11.6	1.88	71.51	2.7	2152	1	28	0	2.75	204
pasta mix, italian four chs lasagna, unprep	1 cup	355	12.53	2.7	70.26	2.6	2093	1	55		3.12	271
pasta mix, italian lasagna, unprep	1 cup	356	10.9	1.97	73.77	2.8	1850	1	52	0	2.87	277
pasta w/ tomato sau, no meat, cnd	1 cup	70	2.22	0.44	14.22	0.9	272	1	13	0	0.91	192
pasta w/sliced franks in tomato sau, cnd entree	1 cup	90	4.37	2.38	12.7	1.6	287	9	60	16	0.91	191
pasta, ckd, enr, w/ added salt	1 cup, spaghetti not packed	157	5.8	0.93	30.59	1.8	131	0	7	0	1.28	44
pasta, ckd, enr, wo/ added salt	1 cup, spaghetti not packed	158	5.8	0.93	30.86	1.8	1	0	7	0	1.28	44
pasta, ckd, unenr, w/ added salt	1 cup, spaghetti not packed	157	5.8	0.93	30.59	1.8	131	0	7	0	0.5	44
pasta, ckd, unenr, wo/ added salt	1 cup, spaghetti not packed	158	5.8	0.93	30.86	1.8	1	0	7	0	0.5	44
pasta, homemade, made w/egg, ckd	2 oz	130	5.28	1.74	23.54		83	41	10		1.16	21
pasta, homemade, made wo/egg, ckd	2 oz	124	4.37	0.98	25.12		74	0	6		1.13	19
pasta, whl grain, 51% whl wheat, remaining enr semolina, ckd	1 cup, spaghetti not packed	156	5.67	1.48	30.87	4.5	4		11		1.58	71
pasta, whl grain, 51% whl wheat, remaining unenr semolina, ckd	1 cup, spaghetti not packed	159	5.82	1.5	31.51	4.6	6		12		1.65	77
pasta, whole-wheat, ckd	1 cup, spaghetti not packed	149	5.99	1.71	30.07	3.9	4	0	13	0	1.72	96
pastrami bf 98% fat-free	1 serving, 6 slices	95	19.6	1.16	1.54	0	1010	47	9		2.78	228
pastrami, turkey	2 slices	139	16.3	6.21	3.34	0.1	1123	68	11	10	4.2	345
peaall types, ckd, bld, w/salt	1 cup, in shell, edible yield	318	13.5	22.01	21.26	8.8	751	0	55	0	1.01	180
peaall types, dry-roasted, w/salt	1 oz	587	24.35	49.66	21.26	8.4	410	0	58	0	1.58	634
peaches, cnd, ex hvy syrup pk, sol&liquids	1 cup, halves or slices	96	0.47	0.03	26.06	1	8	0	3	0	0.29	83
peaches, cnd, ex lt syrup, sol&liquids	1 cup, halves or slices	42	0.4	0.1	11.1	1	5	0	5	0	0.3	74
peaches, cnd, h2o pk, sol&liquids	1 cup, halves or slices	24	0.44	0.06	6.11	1.3	3	0	2	0	0.32	99
peaches, yel, raw	1 cup, slices	39	0.91	0.25	9.54	1.5	0	0	6	0	0.25	190
peanut bar	1 oz	522	15.5	33.7	47.4	4.1	156	0	78	0	0.97	407
peanut brittle, prepared-from-recipe	1 oz	486	7.57	18.98	71.24	2.5	445	12	27	0	1.22	168
peanut butter w/ omega-3, creamy	1 tbsp	608	24.47	54.17	17	6.1	356		45		1.67	780
peanut butter, chunk style, w/salt	2 tbsp	589	24.06	49.94	21.57	8	486	0	45	0	1.9	745

Food	Serving	Cals	Protein (g)	Fat (g)	Carbs (g)	Fiber (g)	Sodium (mg)	Cholesterol (mg)	Calcium (mg)	Vit D (IU)	Iron (mg)	Potassium (mg)
peanut butter, chunk style, wo/salt	2 tbsp	589	24.06	49.94	21.57	8	17	0	45	0	1.9	745
peanut butter, smooth style, w/ salt	2 tbsp	598	22.21	51.36	22.31	5	426	0	49	0	1.74	558
peanut butter, smooth style, wo/salt	2 tbsp	598	22.21	51.36	22.31	5	17	0	49	0	1.74	558
peanut butter, smooth, red fat	2 tablespoon	520	25.9	34	35.65	5.2	540	0	35	0	1.9	669
peanut flour, defatted	1 cup	327	52.2	0.55	34.7	15.8	180	0	140	0	2.1	1290
peanut flour, low fat	1 cup	428	33.8	21.9	31.27	15.8	1	0	130	0	4.74	1358
peanut sprd, red sugar	2 tbsp	650	24.8	54.89	14.23	7.8	292	0	72	0	2.84	818
pears, asian, raw	1 pear	42	0.5	0.23	10.65	3.6	0	0	4	0	0	121
pears, cnd, ex hvy syrup pk, sol&liquids	1 cup, halves	97	0.19	0.13	25.25	1.6	5	0	5	0	0.22	64
pears, cnd, ex lt syrup pk, sol&liquids	1 cup, halves	47	0.3	0.1	12.2	1.6	2	0	7	0	0.2	45
pears, cnd, h2o pk, sol&liquids	1 cup, halves	29	0.19	0.03	7.81	1.6	2	0	4	0	0.21	53
pears, raw	1 cup, slices	57	0.36	0.14	15.23	3.1	1	0	9	0	0.18	116
peas & carrots, frz, ckd, bld, drnd, wo/salt	10 oz	48	3.09	0.42	10.12	3.1	68	0	23	0	0.94	158
peas, edible-podded, bld, drnd, wo/ salt	1 cup	42	3.27	0.23	7.05	2.8	4	0	42	0	1.97	240
peas, green, raw	1 cup	81	5.42	0.4	14.45	5.7	5	0	25	0	1.47	244
peas, grn (includes baby & lesuer types), cnd, drnd sol, unprep	1 cup	68	4.47	0.8	11.36	4.9	273	0	23	0	1.18	106
peas, rstd, wasabi-flavored	1 cup	432	14.11	14.11	62.2	3.8	300	0	123	0	3.8	732
pecans	1 cup, chopped	691	9.17	71.97	13.86	9.6	0	0	70	0	2.53	410
pecans, dry rstd, w/salt	1 oz	710	9.5	74.27	13.55	9.4	383	0	72	0	2.8	424
pecans, dry rstd, wo/salt	1 oz	710	9.5	74.27	13.55	9.4	1	0	72	0	2.8	424
pepper-type, contains caffeine	1 fl oz	41	0	0.1	10.4	0	10	0	3		0.04	1
pepper, banana, raw	1 cup	27	1.66	0.45	5.35	3.4	13	0	14	0	0.46	256
pepper, black	1 tsp, ground	251	10.39	3.26	63.95	25.3	20	0	443	0	9.71	1329
pepper, red or cayenne	1 tsp	318	12.01	17.27	56.63	27.2	30	0	148	0	7.8	2014
peppermint, fresh	2 leaves	70	3.75	0.94	14.89	8	31	0	243	0	5.08	569
pepperoni, bf & pork, sliced	3 oz	504	19.25	46.28	1.18	0	1582	97	19	52	1.33	274
peppers, ancho, dried	1 pepper	281	11.86	8.2	51.42	21.6	43	0	61	0	10.93	2411
peppers, chili, grn, cnd	1 cup	21	0.72	0.27	4.6	1.7	397	0	36	0	1.33	113
peppers, hot chile, sun-dried	1 cup	324	10.58	5.81	69.86	28.7	91	0	45	0	6.04	1870
peppers, hot chili, grn, cnd, pods, excluding sol&liquids	1 pepper	21	0.9	0.1	5.1	1.3	1173	0	7	0	0.5	187
peppers, hot chili, grn, raw	1 pepper	40	2	0.2	9.46	1.5	7	0	18	0	1.2	340
peppers, hot chili, red, cnd, excluding sol&liquids	1 pepper	21	0.9	0.1	5.1	1.3	1173	0	7	0	0.5	187
peppers, hot chili, red, raw	1 pepper	40	1.87	0.44	8.81	1.5	9	0	14	0	1.03	322
peppers, hot pickled, cnd	.25 cup, drained	22	0.8	0.4	4.56	2.6	1430	0	61	0	0.32	113
peppers, jalapeno, cnd, sol&liquids	1 cup, chopped	27	0.92	0.94	4.74	2.6	1671	0	23	0	1.88	193
peppers, jalapeno, raw	1 cup, sliced	29	0.91	0.37	6.5	2.8	3	0	12	0	0.25	248
peppers, pasilla, dried	1 pepper	345	12.35	15.85	51.13	26.8	89	0	97	0	9.83	2222
peppers, serrano, raw	1 cup, chopped	32	1.74	0.44	6.7	3.7	10	0	11	0	0.86	305
peppers, sweet, yellow, raw	1 pepper	27	1	0.21	6.32	0.9	2	0	11	0	0.46	212
peppers, swt, grn, ckd, bld, drnd, w/salt	1 tbsp	26	0.92	0.2	6.11	1.2	238	0	9	0	0.46	166
peppers, swt, grn, ckd, bld, drnd, wo/salt	1 cup, chopped or strips	28	0.92	0.2	6.7	1.2	2	0	9	0	0.46	166
peppers, swt, grn, cnd, sol&liquids	1 cup, halves	18	0.8	0.3	3.9	1.2	1369	0	41	0	0.8	146
peppers, swt, grn, raw	1 cup, chopped	20	0.86	0.17	4.64	1.7	3	0	10	0	0.34	175
peppers, swt, red, ckd, bld, drnd, w/salt	1 tbsp	26	0.92	0.2	6.11	1.2	238	0	9	0	0.46	166
peppers, swt, red, ckd, bld, drnd, wo/salt	1 cup, strips	28	0.92	0.2	6.7	1.2	2	0	9	0	0.46	166
peppers, swt, red, cnd, sol&liquids	1 cup, halves	18	0.8	0.3	3.9	1.2	1369	0	41	0	0.8	146
peppers, swt, red, raw	1 cup, chopped	31	0.99	0.3	6.03	2.1	4	0	7	0	0.43	211

Food	Serving	Cals	Protein (g)	Fat (g)	Carbs (g)	Fiber (g)	Sodium (mg)	Cholesterol (mg)	Calcium (mg)	Vit D (IU)	Iron (mg)	Potassium (mg)
phyllo dough	1 oz	299	7.1	6	52.6	1.9	483	0	11	0	3.21	74
pickle relish, hamburger	1 tbsp	129	0.63	0.54	34.48	3.2	1096	0	4	0	1.14	76
pickle relish, hot dog	1 tbsp	91	1.5	0.46	23.35	1.5	1091	0	5	0	1.25	78
pickle relish, sweet	1 tbsp	130	0.37	0.47	35.06	1.1	811	0	3	0	0.87	25
pickles, cucumber, dill or kosher dill	1 spear, small	12	0.5	0.3	2.41	1	809	0	57	0	0.26	117
pickles, cucumber, sour	1 cup	11	0.33	0.2	2.26	1.2	1208	0	0	0	0.4	23
pickles, cucumber, swt (includes bread & butter pickles)	1 cup, chopped	91	0.58	0.41	21.15	1	457	0	61	0	0.25	100
pie crust, cookie-type, choc, ready crust	1 crust	484	6.08	22.42	64.48	2.7	503	0	32	0	4.3	187
pie crust, cookie-type, graham cracker, ready crust	1 oz	501	5.1	24.83	64.3	1.9	471	0	29	0	2.6	113
pie crust, cookie-type, prep fr recipe, graham cracker, chilled	1 piece	484	4.1	24.4	63.9	1.5	560	0	20		2.12	86
pie crust, cookie-type, prep from recipe, vanilla wafer, chilled	1 cup	531	3.7	36.2	50.2	0.1	515	39	42	21	1.63	79
pie crust, deep dish, frz, bkd, made w/ enr flr	1 pie crust	521	6.1	31.84	52.47	2.3	393		23		2.47	103
pie crust, deep dish, frz, unbaked, made w/ enr flr	1 pie crust	468	5.52	28.74	46.79	1.4	353		20		2.26	91
pie crust, refr, reg, bkd	1 pie crust	506	3.41	28.69	58.52	1.4	472		12		1.15	83
pie crust, standard-type, dry mix, prep, bkd	1 piece	501	6.7	30.4	50.4	1.8	729	0	60		2.15	62
pie crust, standard-type, frz, rtb, enr, bkd	1 pie crust	508	6.5	28.59	56.24	3.3	467	0	21	0	2.8	114
pie crust, standard-type, prep from recipe, bkd	1 piece	527	6.4	34.6	47.5	1.7	542	0	10		2.89	67
pie fillings, appl, cnd	.125 can	100	0.1	0.1	26.1	1	47	0	4	0	0.29	45
pie fillings, blueberry, cnd	.125 can	181	0.41	0.2	44.38	2.6	12	0	27	0	0.8	115
pie fillings, cherry, lo cal	.125 can	53	0.82	0.16	11.98	1.2	12	0	11	0	0.33	118
pie fillings, cnd, cherry	.125 can	115	0.37	0.07	28	0.6	18	0	11	0	0.24	105
pie, appl, commly prep, enr flr	1 oz	237	1.9	11	34	1.6	201	0	11	0	0.45	65
pie, appl, commly prep, unenr flr	1 oz	237	1.9	11	34	1.6	266	0	11		1.21	65
pie, appl, prep from recipe	1 oz	265	2.4	12.5	37.1		211	0	7		1.12	79
pie, banana crm, prep from mix, no-bake type	1 oz	251	3.4	12.9	31.6	0.6	290	29	73		0.46	113
pie, banana crm, prep from recipe	1 oz	269	4.4	13.6	32.9	0.7	240	51	75	32	1.04	165
pie, blueberry, commly prep	1 oz	232	1.8	10	34.9	1	287	0	8	0	0.3	50
pie, blueberry, prep from recipe	1 oz	245	2.7	11.9	33.5		185	0	7		1.23	50
pie, cherry, commly prep	1 oz	260	2	11	39.8	0.8	246	0	12	0	0.48	81
pie, cherry, prep from recipe	1 oz	270	2.8	12.2	38.5		191	0	10		1.85	77
pie, choc creme, commly prep	1 oz	353	4.15	22.41	38.44	0.8	266	12	66	3	1.49	161
pie, choc mousse, prep from mix, no-bake type	1 oz	260	3.5	15.4	29.6		460	35	77		1.08	285
pie, cocnt creme, commly prep	1 oz	298	2.1	16.6	37.3	1.3	204	0	29	6	0.8	65
pie, cocnt crm, prep from mix, no-bake type	1 oz	276	2.8	17.6	28.5	0.5	329	23	72		0.4	141
pie, cocnt custard, commly prep	1 oz	260	5.9	13.2	30.2	1.8	335	35	81		0.8	175
pie, dutch appl, commly prep	1 oz	290	2.17	11.5	44.54	1.6	200	0	14		0.91	76
pie, egg custard, commly prep	1 oz	210	5.5	11.6	20.8	1.6	275	33	80	34	0.58	106
pie, fried pies, cherry	1 oz	316	3	16.1	42.6	2.6	374	0	22		1.22	65
pie, fried pies, fruit	1 oz	316	3	16.1	42.6	2.6	333	0	22	0	1.22	65
pie, fried pies, lemon	1 oz	316	3	16.1	42.6	2.6	374	0	22		1.22	65
pie, lemon meringue, commly prep	1 oz	268	1.5	8.7	47.2	1.2	172	45	56	7	0.61	89
pie, lemon meringue, prep from recipe	1 oz	285	3.8	12.9	39.1		242	53	12		1	65
pie, mince, prep from recipe	1 oz	289	2.6	10.8	48	2.6	254	0	22	0	1.49	203
pie, peach	1 oz	224	1.9	10	32.9	0.8	217	0	8	0	0.5	125
pie, pecan, commly prep	1 oz	407	4.5	16.69	59.61	2.1	275	42	22	3	0.93	99
pie, pecan, prep from recipe	1 oz	412	4.9	22.2	52.2		262	87	32		1.48	133
pie, pumpkin, commly prep	1 oz	243	3.9	9.75	34.83	1.8	239	26	64	2	0.9	167
pie, pumpkin, prep from recipe	1 oz	204	4.5	9.3	26.4		225	42	94		1.27	186
pie, vanilla crm, prep from recipe	1 oz	278	4.8	14.4	32.6	0.6	260	62	90	47	1.02	126
pike, northern, ckd, dry heat	3 oz	113	24.69	0.88	0	0	49	50	73		0.71	331
pike, northern, liver (alaska native)	3 oz	156	16.6	8	4.3				28		2.1	

Food	Serving	Cals	Protein (g)	Fat (g)	Carbs (g)	Fiber (g)	Sodium (mg)	Cholesterol (mg)	Calcium (mg)	Vit D (IU)	Iron (mg)	Potassium (mg)
pike, walleye, ckd, dry heat	1 fillet	119	24.54	1.56	0	0	65	110	141		1.67	499
pili dried	1 cup	719	10.8	79.55	3.98		3	0	145		3.53	507
pimento, canned	1 tbsp	23	1.1	0.3	5.1	1.9	14	0	6	0	1.68	158
pine dried	1 cup	673	13.69	68.37	13.08	3.7	2	0	16	0	5.53	597
pine pinyon, dried	1 oz	629	11.57	60.98	19.3	10.7	72	0	8	0	3.06	628
pineapple & grapefruit juc drk, cnd	1 fl oz	47	0.2	0.1	11.6	0.1	14	0	7	0	0.31	61
pineapple & orange juc drk, cnd	1 fl oz	50	1.3	0	11.8	0.1	3	0	5	0	0.27	46
pineapple juc, cnd or btld, unswtnd, w/ added vit c	1 cup	53	0.36	0.12	12.87	0.2	2	0	13	0	0.31	130
pineapple juc, frz conc, unswtnd, undil	1 can	179	1.3	0.1	44.3	0.7	3	0	39	0	0.9	472
pineapple, cnd, ex hvy syrup pk, sol&liquids	1 cup, crushed, sliced, or chunks	83	0.34	0.11	21.5	0.8	1	0	14	0	0.38	102
pineapple, cnd, h2o pk, sol&liquids	1 cup, crushed, sliced, or chunks	32	0.43	0.09	8.3	0.8	1	0	15	0	0.4	127
pineapple, cnd, lt syrup pk, sol&liquids	1 cup, crushed, sliced, or chunks	52	0.36	0.12	13.45	0.8	1	0	14	0	0.39	105
pineapple, raw, all var	1 cup, chunks	50	0.54	0.12	13.12	1.4	1	0	13	0	0.29	109
pistachio dry rstd, w/salt	1 cup	569	21.05	45.82	27.55	10.3	428	0	107	0	4.03	1007
pistachio dry rstd, wo/salt	1 cup	572	21.05	45.82	28.28	10.3	6	0	107	0	4.03	1007
pistachio raw	1 cup	560	20.16	45.32	27.17	10.6	1	0	105	0	3.92	1025
pita chips, salted	1 oz	457	11.79	15.2	68.26	3.8	854	0	17	0	4.59	129
pizza chain, 14" pizza, chs topping, reg crust	1 slice	266	11.39	9.69	33.33	2.3	598	17	188	0	2.48	172
pizza chain, 14" pizza, chs topping, stuffed crust	1 slice	274	12.23	11.63	30	1.7	615	30	238	0	2.04	229
pizza chain, 14" pizza, chs topping, thick crust	1 slice	271	10.81	10.54	33.17	2.2	597	17	179	0	2.48	169
pizza chain, 14" pizza, chs topping, thin crust	1 slice	302	12.85	13.95	31.2	2.5	742	28	288	0	1.71	199
pizza chain, 14" pizza, meat & veg topping, reg crust	1 slice	244	11.02	10.9	25.38	2.2	589	27	120	0	1.86	184
pizza chain, 14" pizza, pepperoni topping, reg crust	1 slice	282	11.74	11.91	31.98	2.3	685	25	153	0	2.52	195
pizza chain, 14" pizza, pepperoni topping, thick crust	1 slice	287	11.49	12.58	31.84	2.2	684	24	148	0	2.55	189
pizza chain, 14" pizza, pepperoni topping, thin crust	1 slice	331	14.01	17.61	29	2.3	875	37	216	0	1.95	223
pizza chain, 14" pizza, sausage topping, reg crust	1 slice	280	11.5	12.35	30.62	2.3	633	23	144	0	2.41	197
pizza chain, 14" pizza, sausage topping, thick crust	1 slice	282	11.06	12.94	30.36	2.3	637	23	143	0	2.45	190
pizza chain, 14" pizza, sausage topping, thin crust	1 slice	321	13.36	17.71	27	2.5	782	36	213	0	1.73	225
pizza rolls, frz, unprep	6 rolls	328	8.73	9.98	50.72	1.2	599	6	125	1	1.8	301
pizza, chs topping, reg crust, frz, ckd	9 servings per 24 oz package	268	10.36	12.28	29.02	2.2	447	14	179	0	2.27	152
pizza, chs topping, rising crust, frz, ckd	6 servings per 29.25 oz package	260	12.37	8.78	32.91	2.5	556	16	177	0	1.77	175
pizza, chs topping, thin crust, frz, ckd	1 slice	263	11.91	11.07	28.8	3	471	21	228	0	2.14	201
pizza, meat & veg topping, reg crust, frz, ckd	5 servings per 24.2 oz package	276	11.28	14.43	25.14	2.2	555	16	152	0	1.36	209
pizza, meat & veg topping, rising crust, frz, ckd	6 servings per 34.98 oz package	271	12.63	11.75	28.78	2.3	640	19	155	0	1.36	189
pizza, meat topping, thick crust, frz, ckd	1 slice	274	11.76	11.52	30.76	2.3	690	21	150	0	1.7	201

Food	Serving	Cals	Protein (g)	Fat (g)	Carbs (g)	Fiber (g)	Sodium (mg)	Cholesterol (mg)	Calcium (mg)	Vit D (IU)	Iron (mg)	Potassium (mg)
pizza, pepperoni topping, reg crust, frz, ckd	.25 pizza, 12" diameter	274	14.38	13.13	24.69	2	590	27	168	0	2.43	239
plantain chips, salted	1 oz	531	2.28	29.59	63.84	3.5	202	0	9	0	0.97	786
plantains, cooked	1 cup, mashed	116	0.79	0.18	31.15	2.3	5	0	2	0	0.58	465
plantains, grn, fried	1 cup	309	1.5	11.81	49.17	3.5	2		4		0.67	482
plantains, raw	1 cup, sliced	122	1.3	0.37	31.89	2.3	4	0	3	0	0.6	499
plantains, yel, fried, latino restaurant	1 cup	236	1.42	7.51	40.77	3.2	6		6		0.62	507
plums, dried (prunes), unckd	1 cup, pitted	240	2.18	0.38	63.88	7.1	2	0	43	0	0.93	732
plums, raw	1 cup, sliced	46	0.7	0.28	11.42	1.4	0	0	6	0	0.17	157
polish sausage, pork	3 oz	326	14.1	28.72	1.63	0	876	70	12		1.44	237
pollock, alaska, ckd (not previously frozen)	3 oz	80	19.42	0.26	0		166	74	13		0.29	364
pollock, alaska, ckd, dry heat (maybe previously frozen)	1 fillet	111	23.48	1.18	0	0	419	86	72	51	0.56	430
pollock, atlantic, ckd, dry heat	3 oz	118	24.92	1.26	0	0	110	91	77		0.59	456
pomegranate juc, bttld	1 cup	54	0.15	0.29	13.13	0.1	9	0	11	0	0.1	214
pomegranates, raw	.5 cup, arils	83	1.67	1.17	18.7	4	3	0	10	0	0.3	236
pompano, florida, ckd, dry heat	1 fillet	211	23.69	12.14	0	0	76	64	43		0.67	636
popcorn, air-popped	1 cup	387	12.94	4.54	77.78	14.5	8	0	7	0	3.19	329
popcorn, microwav, regula (butter) flavo, mad with pal oil	1 cup	535	8.38	30.22	57.26	10	763	0	23	0	2.06	393
popcorn, microwave, lofat&na	1 oz	429	12.6	9.5	73.39	14.2	490	0	11	0	2.28	241
pork & bf sausage, frsh, ckd	1 link	396	13.8	36.25	2.7	0	929	71	10	28	1.13	189
pork & turkey sausage, pre-cooked	1 serving	342	12.05	30.64	3.63	0	876	72	74		1.3	230
pork loin, frsh, backribs, bone-in, cooked-roasted, ln	3 oz	255	24.15	17.65	0	0	98	84	44	46	0.96	249
pork sausage rice links, brown&serve, ckd	2 links	407	13.7	37.63	2.36	0	689	66	15	36	1.12	212
pork sausage, link/patty, ckd, pan-fried	1 patty	325	18.53	27.25	1.42	0	814	86	9	58	1.2	342
pork sausage, link/patty, fully ckd, microwaved	1 patty	438	15.12	41.66	0.62	0	990	79	17	41	0.95	225
pork sausage, link/patty, fully ckd, unhtd	1 link	392	13.46	37.25	0.69	0	810	74	16	48	0.92	211
pork sausage, link/patty, red fat, ckd, pan-fried	3 oz	267	20.94	20.32	0.15	0	698	82	19	58	1.91	328
pork sausage, red na, ckd	3 oz	271	9.41	22.35	8.13	0	294	59	0	30	0.85	160
pork skins, barbecue-flavor	1 oz	538	57.9	31.8	1.6		2667	115	43		1.04	180
pork skins, plain	1 oz	544	61.3	31.3	0	0	1818	95	30	0	0.88	127
pork, bacon, rendered fat, ckd	3 oz	898	0.07	99.5	0	0	27	97	1		0.13	15
pork, cured, bacon, ckd, bkd	1 slice, cooked	548	35.73	43.27	1.35	0	2193	107	10		1.49	539
pork, cured, bacon, ckd, brld, pan-fried or rstd, red na	1 slice, cooked	541	37.04	41.78	1.43	0	1030	110	11	42	1.44	565
pork, cured, bacon, ckd, microwaved	1 slice, cooked	476	39.01	34.12	0.48	0	1783	111	13		1.14	525
pork, cured, bacon, pre-sliced, ckd, pan-fried	1 slice	468	33.92	35.09	1.7	0	1684	99	11	17	0.95	499
pork, cured, fat (from ham&arm picnic), rstd	1 oz	591	7.64	61.86	0	0	624	86	8		0.61	164
pork, cured, feet, pickled	1 oz	140	11.63	10.02	0.01	0	946	83	32	16	0.31	13
pork, cured, ham -- h2o added, rump, bone-in, ln & fat, htd, rstd	3 oz	161	20.1	8.56	0.99	0	1101	63	8		0.69	244
pork, cured, ham -- h2o added, shank, bone-in, ln & fat, htd, rstd	3 oz	200	18.62	13.37	1.35	0	988	66	9		1.37	232
pork, cured, ham -- h2o added, slce, bne-in, ln & fat, htd, pan-brl	3 oz	166	20.8	8.73	1.54	0	1309	66	11		1.07	280
pork, cured, ham -- h2o added, whl, bnless, ln & fat, htd, rstd	3 oz	126	17.77	5.48	1.54	0	1181	54	9	29	0.82	313
pork, cured, ham & h2o prdct, slce, bne-in, ln & fat, htd, pan-brl	3 oz	155	19.85	7.78	1.41	0	1188	64	11		0.9	281
pork, cured, ham & h2o prdct, slice, bnless, ln & fat, htd, pan-brl	1 slice	124	15.08	5.13	4.69	0	1389	45	8	34	0.74	272

Food	Serving	Cals	Protein (g)	Fat (g)	Carbs (g)	Fiber (g)	Sodium (mg)	Cholesterol (mg)	Calcium (mg)	Vit D (IU)	Iron (mg)	Potassium (mg)
pork, cured, ham & h2o product, rump, bone-in, ln & fat, htd, rstd	3 oz	186	19.46	11.48	1.15	0	1181	67	10		0.82	254
pork, cured, ham & h2o product, shank, bone-in, ln & fat, htd, rstd	3 oz	234	18.17	17.29	1.42	0	945	72	8		1	216
pork, cured, ham & h2o product, slice, bnless, ln, htd, pan-broil	1 slice	123	15.09	5.06	4.69	0	1390	45	8	34	0.74	272
pork, cured, ham & h2o product, whl, bnless, ln & fat, htd, rstd	3 oz	123	13.88	5.46	4.61	0	1335	43	8	27	0.74	245
pork, cured, ham w/ nat jucs, sprl slce, bnles, ln & fat, htd, rstd	1 slice	139	22.18	5.1	1.06	0	977	64	4	33	0.83	345
pork, cured, ham w/ nat juices, rump, bone-in, ln & fat, htd, rstd	3 oz	177	22.47	9.39	0.6	0	841	72	10		0.99	477
pork, ground, 72% ln / 28% fat, ckd, crumbles	4 oz	393	22.83	32.93	1.39	0	94	100	20	34	1.15	280
pork, ground, 72% ln / 28% fat, ckd, pan-broiled	3 oz, grilled patties	377	22.59	31.42	1.08	0	91	99	20	32	1.21	275
pork, ground, 84% ln / 16% fat, ckd, crumbles	3 oz, grilled patties	289	26.69	20.04	0.58	0	89	89	20	20	1.1	354
pork, ground, 84% ln / 16% fat, ckd, pan-broiled	3 oz, grilled patties	301	27.14	21.39	0	0	89	97	20	22	1.16	345
pork, ground, 84% ln / 16% fat, raw	4 oz	218	17.99	16	0.44	0	68	68	15	17	0.88	244
pork, ground, 96% ln / 4% fat, ckd, crumbles	3 oz, grilled patties	187	30.55	7.15	0	0	84	78	19	7	1.05	428
pork, ground, 96% ln / 4% fat, ckd, pan-broiled	3 oz, grilled patties	185	31.69	6.2	0.57	0	88	85	20	6	1.11	415
pork, ground, 96% ln / 4% fat, raw	4 oz	121	21.1	4	0.21	0	67	59	15	4	0.86	310
potato chips, barbecue-flavor	1 oz	487	6.51	31.06	55.92	3.8	545	0	32	0	1.36	1186
potato chips, cheese-flavor	1 oz	496	8.5	27.2	57.7	5.2	458	4	72		1.84	1528
potato chips, fat free, salted	1 oz	379	9.64	0.6	83.76	7.5	643	0	35	0	3.57	1628
potato chips, fr dried potatoes, multigrain	1 oz	505	5.3	24.74	65.34	2.7	544	0	26	0	0.85	330
potato chips, fr dried potatoes, sour-cream & onion-flavor	1 oz	547	6.6	37	51.3	1.2	541	3	64		1.4	496
potato chips, from dried potatoes, cheese-flavor	1 oz	551	7	37	50.6	3.4	600	4	110		1.6	381
potato chips, from dried potatoes, lt	1 oz	502	4.56	26.14	64.76	3.2	450	0	29	0	1.11	760
potato chips, from dried potatoes, pln	1 oz	545	4.62	35.28	55.38	2.9	400	0	17	0	0.8	637
potato chips, plain, salted	1 oz	532	6.39	33.98	53.83	3.1	527	0	21	0	1.28	1196
potato chips, pln, made w/part hydr soybn oil, salted	1 oz	536	7	34.6	52.9	4.8	594	0	24		1.63	1275
potato chips, pln, made w/part hydr soybn oil, unsalted	1 oz	536	7	34.6	52.9	4.8	8	0	24		1.63	1275
potato chips, pln, unsalted	1 oz	536	7	34.6	52.9	4.8	8	0	24	0	1.63	1275
potato chips, sour-cream-and-onion-flavor	1 oz	531	8.1	33.9	51.5	5.2	549	7	72		1.6	1331
potato chips, white, restructured, bkd	1 cup	469	5	18.2	71.4	4.8	554	0	125	0	0.8	721
potato chips, wo/salt, red fat	1 oz	487	7.1	20.8	67.8	6.1	8	0	21	0	1.35	1744
potato flour	1 cup	357	6.9	0.34	83.1	5.9	55	0	65	0	1.38	1001
potato pancakes	1 pancake	268	6.08	14.76	27.81	3.3	764	95	32	11	1.67	622
potato puffs, frz, oven-heated	10 puffs	192	2.13	9.05	27.29	2	463	0	14	0	0.58	287
potato puffs, frz, unprep	1 cup	178	1.93	8.71	24.8	2.3	428	0	13	0	0.47	247
potato salad	.333 cup	114	1.53	6.03	13.53		328	60	14		0.73	270
potato salad w/ egg	.5 cup	157	1.96	9.4	16.18	1.3	329	17	15	4	0.5	242
potato salad, home-prepared	1 cup	143	2.68	8.2	11.17	1.3	529	68	19	0	0.65	254
potato soup, inst, dry mix	1/3 cup	343	9.2	3.1	76.14	7.6	2400	12	172	0	2.38	1248
potato, frnch fried in veg oil, fast food	1 serving, small	312	3.43	14.73	41.44	3.8	210	0	18	0	0.81	579
potato, mashed	1 cup	89	1.65	2.82	14.65	1.3	306	0	18	0	0.31	286
potato\, yel flsh, hash brn, shrd, salt added in proc, frz, unprep	3 oz	81	2.04	0.07	17.98	2	330	0	9		0.31	398
potatoes, au gratin, dry mix, prep w/ h2o, whl milk&butter	5.5 oz	93	2.3	4.12	12.84	0.9	439	15	83		0.32	219
potatoes, au gratin, dry mix, unprep	5.5 oz	314	8.9	3.7	74.31	4.1	2095		311	0	1.63	990
potatoes, au gratin, home-prepared from recipe using butter	1 cup	132	5.06	7.59	11.27	1.8	433	23	119	0	0.64	396

Food	Serving	Cals	Protein (g)	Fat (g)	Carbs (g)	Fiber (g)	Sodium (mg)	Cholesterol (mg)	Calcium (mg)	Vit D (IU)	Iron (mg)	Potassium (mg)
potatoes, au gratin, home-prepared from recipe using margarine	1 cup	132	5.06	7.59	11.27	1.8	433	15	119	0	0.64	396
potatoes, bkd, flesh & skn, w/ salt	.5 cup	93	2.5	0.13	21.15	2.2	10	0	15	0	1.08	535
potatoes, bkd, flesh & skn, wo/ salt	.5 cup	93	2.5	0.13	21.15	2.2	10	0	15	0	1.08	535
potatoes, bkd, flesh, w/salt	.5 cup	93	1.96	0.1	21.55	1.5	241	0	5	0	0.35	391
potatoes, bkd, flesh, wo/salt	.5 cup	93	1.96	0.1	21.55	1.5	5	0	5	0	0.35	391
potatoes, bkd, skn only, w/ salt	1 skin	198	4.29	0.1	46.06	7.9	257	0	34	0	7.04	573
potatoes, bkd, skn, wo/salt	1 skin	198	4.29	0.1	46.06	7.9	21	0	34	0	7.04	573
potatoes, bld, ckd in skn, flesh, w/salt	.5 cup	87	1.87	0.1	20.13	2	240	0	5	0	0.31	379
potatoes, bld, ckd in skn, flesh, wo/salt	.5 cup	87	1.87	0.1	20.13	1.8	4	0	5	0	0.31	379
potatoes, bld, ckd in skn, skn, w/salt	1 skin	78	2.86	0.1	17.2	3.3	250	0	45	0	6.07	407
potatoes, bld, ckd in skn, skn, wo/salt	1 skin	78	2.86	0.1	17.21	3.3	14	0	45	0	6.07	407
potatoes, bld, ckd wo/ skn, flesh, w/ salt	.5 cup	86	1.71	0.1	20.01	2	241	0	8	0	0.31	328
potatoes, bld, ckd wo/ skn, flesh, wo/ salt	.5 cup	86	1.71	0.1	20.01	1.8	5	0	8	0	0.31	328
potatoes, cnd, drnd sol	1 cup	60	1.41	0.21	13.61	2.3	219	0	5	0	1.26	229
potatoes, cnd, drnd sol, no salt	1 cup	62	1.4	0.2	13.6	2.4	5	0	5	0	1.26	229
potatoes, cnd, sol&liquids	1 cup, whole	44	1.2	0.11	9.89	1.4	217	0	39	0	0.72	205
potatoes, flesh & skn, raw	.5 cup, diced	77	2.05	0.09	17.49	2.1	6	0	12	0	0.81	425
potatoes, fr fr, all types, salt not added in proc, frz, as purch	10 strips	150	2.24	4.66	24.81	1.9	23	0	9	0	0.62	408
potatoes, fr fr, all types, salt not added in proc, frz, ovn-htd	10 strip	172	2.66	5.22	28.71	2.6	32	0	12	0	0.74	451
potatoes, fr fr, crnkl or reg, salt added in proc, frz, as purch	10 strip	150	2.34	4.99	23.96	2	349	0	13	0	0.62	380
potatoes, fr fr, crnkl/reg cut, salt added in proc, frz, oven-htd	10 strip	166	2.51	5.13	27.5	2.3	391	0	13	0	0.75	471
potatoes, french fr, all types, salt added in proc, frz, oven htd	10 fries	158	2.75	5.48	25.55	2	324	0	12	0	0.57	478
potatoes, hash brown, home-prepared	1 cup	265	3	12.52	35.11	3.2	342	0	14	0	0.55	576
potatoes, hash browns, rnd pieces or patty	1 round piece	272	2.58	17.04	28.88	2.7	566	0	19	0	0.6	355
potatoes, scallpd, dry mix, prep w/h2o, whl milk&butter	1 cup, (unprepared)	93	2.12	4.3	12.77	1.1	341	11	36	0	0.38	203
potatoes, scallpd, dry mix, unprep	5.5 oz	358	7.77	4.59	73.93	8.6	1578	5	62	0	2.01	905
potatoes, scallpd, home-prepared w/butter	1 cup	88	2.87	3.68	10.78	1.9	335	12	57	0	0.57	378
potatoes, scallpd, home-prepared w/ margarine	1 cup	88	2.87	3.68	10.78	1.9	335	6	57	0	0.57	378
praline, prepared-from-recipe	1 piece	485	3.3	25.9	59.59	3.5	48	0	43		1.29	217
pretzels, hard, confectioner's coating, chocolate-flavor	1 oz	457	7.5	16.7	70.9	2.4	569	0	74	0	2	225
pretzels, hard, pln, made w/unenr flr, salted	1 oz	381	9.1	3.5	79.2	2.8	1715	0	36		1.67	146
pretzels, hard, pln, made w/unenr flr, unsalted	1 oz	381	9.1	3.5	79.2	2.8	289	0	36		1.67	146
pretzels, hard, pln, salted	1 oz	384	10.04	2.93	80.39	3.4	1240	0	27	0	4.58	223
pretzels, soft	1 large	338	8.2	3.1	69.39	1.7	545	0	23	0	3.92	88
pretzels, soft, unsalted	1 large	345	8.2	3.1	71.04	1.7	252	0	23	0	3.92	88
prickly pears, brld (northern plains indians)	1 pad	91	0.39	0.31	21.57							
protein pdr soy bsd	1 scoop	388	55.56	5.56	28.89	6.7	733	0	178	0	12	933
protein pdr whey bsd	3.5 oz	352	78.13	1.56	6.25	3	156	16	469	0	1.13	500
pudding, choc, dry mix, reg	3.5 oz	362	2.6	2.1	89.3	4.5	479	0	53	0	1.82	209
pudding, cocnt crm, dry mix, inst	3.5 oz	415	0.9	10	83.5	4	1040	0	8	0	0.72	96
puddings, all flavors xcpt choc, lo cal, inst, dry mix	3.5 oz	350	0.81	0.9	84.66	0.8	3750	0	143	0	0.38	30
puddings, all flavors xcpt choc, lo cal, reg, dry mix	3.5 oz	351	1.6	0.1	86.04	0.9	1765	0	49	0	0.05	18
puddings, choc flavor, lo cal, inst, dry mix	3.5 oz	356	5.3	2.4	78.2	6.1	2838	0	126	0	3.11	1279
puddings, choc flavor, lo cal, reg, dry mix	3.5 oz	365	10.08	3	74.42	10.1	3326	0	50	0	3.87	570
puddings, choc, dry mix, inst	3.5 oz	378	2.3	1.9	87.9	3.6	1771	0	12	0	1.29	236

Food	Serving	Cals	Protein (g)	Fat (g)	Carbs (g)	Fiber (g)	Sodium (mg)	Cholesterol (mg)	Calcium (mg)	Vit D (IU)	Iron (mg)	Potassium (mg)
puddings, choc, dry mix, inst, prep w/ 2% milk	.5 cup	105	3.15	1.92	18.89	0.4	284	6	104	33	0.4	168
puddings, choc, dry mix, inst, prep w/ whl milk	.5 cup	111	3.1	3.1	18.8	1	284	11	102		0.29	166
puddings, choc, dry mix, inst, prep w/ whole milk	.5 cup	120	3.16	3.15	19.64	0.8	98	9	106	44	0.34	150
puddings, choc, dry mix, reg, prep w/ 2% milk	.5 cup	111	3.28	2.06	19.76	0.8	102	7	112	42	0.34	156
puddings, rice, ready-to-eat	1 cup	108	3.23	2.15	18.39	0.3	97	12	95	0	0.11	125
puddings, tapioca, dry mix	3.5 oz	369	0.1	0.1	94.3	0.2	477	0	4	0	0.12	5
puddings, tapioca, dry mix, prep w/ 2% milk	.5 cup	105	2.88	1.67	19.56	0	121	6	105	34	0.06	133
puddings, tapioca, dry mix, prep w/ whl milk	.5 cup	115	2.84	2.89	19.43	0	120	12	103	34	0.06	131
puddings, tapioca, dry mix, w/ no added salt	3.5 oz	369	0.1	0.1	94.3	0.2	8	0	4		0.12	5
puddings, tapioca, rte	1 oz	130	1.95	3.88	21.69	0	145	1	71	0	0.11	92
puff pastry, frz, rtb	1 oz	551	7.3	38.1	45.1	1.5	249	0	10		2.56	61
puff pastry, frz, rtb, bkd	1 oz	558	7.4	38.5	45.7	1.5	253	0	10	0	2.6	62
puffs or twists, corn-based, extrdd, cheese-flavor, unenr	1 oz	558	5.76	35.76	54.1	2.2	896	4	58	0	1.1	197
pulled pork in barbecue sau	1 cup	168	13.19	4.42	18.74	1.2	666	35	44	8	1.24	305
pumpkin pie mix, canned	1 cup	104	1.09	0.13	26.39	8.3	208	0	37	0	1.06	138
pumpkin pie spice	1 tsp	342	5.76	12.6	69.28	14.8	52	0	682	0	19.71	663
pumpkin, canned, with salt	1 cup	34	1.1	0.28	8.09	2.9	241	0	26	0	1.39	206
pumpkin, ckd, bld, drnd, w/salt	1 cup, mashed	18	0.72	0.07	4.31	1.1	237	0	15	0	0.57	230
pumpkin, ckd, bld, drnd, wo/salt	1 cup, mashed	20	0.72	0.07	4.9	1.1	1	0	15	0	0.57	230
pumpkin, cnd, wo/salt	1 cup	34	1.1	0.28	8.09	2.9	5	0	26	0	1.39	206
quesadilla, w/ chick	1 quesadilla	294	15.05	15.25	24.04	1.7	745	37	269	8	1.77	183
quinoa, ckd	1 cup	120	4.4	1.92	21.3	2.8	7	0	17	0	1.49	172
quinoa, unckd	1 cup	368	14.12	6.07	64.16	7	5	0	47	0	4.57	563
radicchio, raw	1 cup, shredded	23	1.43	0.25	4.48	0.9	22	0	19	0	0.57	302
radishes, oriental, ckd, bld, drnd, w/salt	1 cup, slices	17	0.67	0.24	3.43	1.6	249	0	17	0	0.15	285
radishes, oriental, ckd, bld, drnd, wo/salt	1 cup, sliced	17	0.67	0.24	3.43	1.6	13	0	17	0	0.15	285
radishes, oriental, raw	1 cup, slices	18	0.6	0.1	4.1	1.6	21	0	27	0	0.4	227
radishes, raw	1 cup, slices	16	0.68	0.1	3.4	1.6	39	0	25	0	0.34	233
raisins, seeded	1 cup, packed	296	2.52	0.54	78.47	6.8	28	0	28	0	2.59	825
raisins, seedless	1 cup, packed	299	3.07	0.46	79.18	3.7	11	0	50	0	1.88	749
raspberries, raw	1 cup	52	1.2	0.65	11.94	6.5	1	0	25	0	0.69	151
ravioli, cheese-filled, cnd	1 cup	77	2.48	1.45	13.64	1.3	306	3	33	0	0.74	232
ravioli, chs w/ tomato sau, frz, not prep, incl reg & lt entrees	1 cup	111	4.52	2.61	17.31	1.4	280	11	79	3	0.93	233
ravioli, meat-filled, w/ tomato sau or meat sau, cnd	1 cup	97	3.24	3.41	13.26	1.5	283	5	12	0	1.09	178
red sugar, cola, contains caffeine & sweeteners	1 fl oz	20	0	0	5.16	0	4	0	2	0	0.02	3
refried bns, cnd, fat-free	1 cup	79	5.34	0.45	13.5	4.7	438	0	34	0	1.62	344
rhubarb, frz, ckd, w/sugar	1 cup	116	0.39	0.05	31.2	2	1	0	145	0	0.21	96
rhubarb, raw	1 cup, diced	21	0.9	0.2	4.54	1.8	4	0	86	0	0.22	288
rice (sake)	1 fl oz	134	0.5	0	5	0	2	0	5	0	0.1	25
rice cakes, brown rice, buckwheat	1 cake	380	9	3.5	80.1	3.8	116	0	11		1.14	299
rice cakes, brown rice, buckwheat, unsalted	1 cake	380	9	3.5	80.1		4	0	11		1.14	299
rice cakes, brown rice, multigrain	1 cake	387	8.5	3.5	80.1	3	252	0	21		1.96	294
rice cakes, brown rice, multigrain, unsalted	1 cake	387	8.5	3.5	80.1		4	0	21		1.96	294
rice cakes, brown rice, pln, unsalted	1 cake	387	8.2	2.8	81.5	4.2	26	0	11	0	1.49	290
rice cakes, brown rice, rye	1 cake	386	8.1	3.8	79.9	4	110	0	21		1.8	311
rice cakes, brown rice, sesame sd	1 cake	392	7.6	3.8	81.5	5.4	227	0	12		1.58	290

Food	Serving	Cals	Protein (g)	Fat (g)	Carbs (g)	Fiber (g)	Sodium (mg)	Cholesterol (mg)	Calcium (mg)	Vit D (IU)	Iron (mg)	Potassium (mg)
rice cakes, brown rice, sesame sd, unsalted	1 cake	392	7.6	3.8	81.5		4	0	12		1.58	290
rice crackers	1 crisp	416	10	5	82.64	0	233	0	0	0	0	243
rice crisps (includes all brands)	1 cup	381	6.45	1.27	86.04	0.7	850		5		10.53	108
rice flour, brown	1 cup	363	7.23	2.78	76.48	4.6	8	0	11	0	1.98	289
rice flr, white, unenr	1 cup	366	5.95	1.42	80.13	2.4	0	0	10	0	0.35	76
rice milk, unswtnd	1 cup	47	0.28	0.97	9.17	0.3	39	0	118	42	0.2	27
rice noodles, ckd	1 cup	108	1.79	0.2	24.01	1	19	0	4	0	0.14	4
rice, brown, long-grain, ckd	1 cup	123	2.74	0.97	25.58	1.6	4	0	3	0	0.56	86
rice, brown, medium-grain, ckd	1 cup	112	2.32	0.83	23.51	1.8	1	0	10	0	0.53	79
rice, white, glutinous, unenr, ckd	1 cup	97	2.02	0.19	21.09	1	5	0	2	0	0.14	10
rice, white, glutinous, unenr, unckd	1 cup	370	6.81	0.55	81.68	2.8	7	0	11	0	1.6	77
rice, white, long-grain, parbld, enr, ckd	1 cup	123	2.91	0.37	26.05	0.9	2	0	19	0	1.81	56
rice, white, long-grain, parbld, enr, dry	1 cup	374	7.51	1.03	80.89	1.8	2	0	71	0	3.33	174
rice, white, long-grain, parbld, unenr, ckd	1 cup	123	2.91	0.37	26.05	0.9	2	0	19	0	0.24	56
rice, white, long-grain, parbld, unenr, dry	1 cup	374	7.51	1.03	80.89	1.8	2	0	71	0	0.74	174
rice, white, long-grain, preckd or inst, enr, dry	1 cup	380	7.82	0.94	82.32	1.9	10	0	22	0	6.3	27
rice, white, long-grain, preckd or inst, enr, prep	1 cup	124	2.18	0.5	26.76	0.6	4	0	8	0	1.77	9
rice, white, long-grain, reg, ckd, enr, w/salt	1 cup	130	2.69	0.28	28.17	0.4	382	0	10	0	1.2	35
rice, white, long-grain, reg, ckd, unenr, w/salt	1 cup	130	2.69	0.28	28.17	0.4	382	0	10	0	0.2	35
rice, white, long-grain, reg, enr, ckd	1 cup	130	2.69	0.28	28.17	0.4	1	0	10	0	1.2	35
rice, white, long-grain, reg, raw, enr	1 cup	365	7.13	0.66	79.95	1.3	5	0	28	0	4.31	115
rice, white, long-grain, reg, raw, unenr	1 cup	365	7.13	0.66	79.95	1.3	5	0	28	0	0.8	115
rice, white, long-grain, reg, unenr, ckd wo/ salt	1 cup	130	2.69	0.28	28.17	0.4	1	0	10	0	0.2	35
rice, white, medium-grain, ckd, unenr	1 cup	130	2.38	0.21	28.59		0	0	3	0	0.2	29
rice, white, medium-grain, enr, ckd	1 cup	130	2.38	0.21	28.59	0.3	0	0	3	0	1.49	29
rice, white, medium-grain, raw, enr	1 cup	360	6.61	0.58	79.34	1.4	1	0	9	0	4.36	86
rice, white, medium-grain, raw, unenr	1 cup	360	6.61	0.58	79.34		1	0	9	0	0.8	86
rice, white, short-grain, ckd, unenr	1 cup	130	2.36	0.19	28.73		0	0	1	0	0.2	26
rice, white, short-grain, enr, ckd	1 cup	130	2.36	0.19	28.73		0	0	1	0	1.46	26
rice, white, short-grain, enr, unckd	1 cup	358	6.5	0.52	79.15	2.8	1	0	3	0	4.23	76
rice, white, short-grain, raw, unenr	1 cup	358	6.5	0.52	79.15		1	0	3	0	0.8	76
rice, white, stmd, chinese restaurant	1 cup, loosely packed	151	3.2	0.27	33.88	0.9	5		5		0.39	20
rich choc, pdr	2 tbsp	372	0	0	92.96	0	636	0	909	364	16.36	0
roast bf sndwch, pln	1 sandwich	244	15.17	10.3	22.21	1.3	653	30	55	1	2.64	224
rolls, dinner, egg	1 roll	307	9.5	6.4	52	3.7	566	50	59	0	3.52	104
rolls, dinner, oat bran	1 roll	236	9.5	4.6	40.2	4.1	413	0	85	0	4.14	121
rolls, dinner, pln, comm prepared (inc brown -n- serve)	1 roll	310	10.86	6.47	52.04	2	467	4	178	0	3.72	139
rolls, dinner, pln, prep from recipe, made w/lofat (2%) milk	1 roll	316	8.5	7.3	53.4	1.9	415	35	60		2.96	152
rolls, dinner, rye	1 roll	286	10.3	3.4	53.1	4.9	650	0	30	0	2.7	180
rolls, dinner, swt	1 roll	321	10.04	7.37	53.58	3.1	253	55	62	0	2.74	149
rolls, dinner, wheat	1 roll	273	8.6	6.3	46	3.8	524	0	176	0	3.55	115
rolls, dinner, whole-wheat	1 roll	266	8.7	4.7	51.1	7.5	521	0	106	0	2.42	272
rolls, french	1 roll	277	8.6	4.3	50.2	3.2	574	0	91	0	2.71	114
rolls, pumpernickel	1 roll	276	10.8	2.8	51.87	5.4	492	0	67	0	2.78	208
root beer	1 fl oz	41	0	0	10.6	0	13	0	5	0	0.05	1
rosemary, dried	1 tsp	331	4.88	15.22	64.06	42.6	50	0	1280	0	29.25	955
rosemary, fresh	1 tsp	131	3.31	5.86	20.7	14.1	26	0	317	0	6.65	668
rutabagas, ckd, bld, drnd, w/salt	.5 cup, mashed	30	0.93	0.18	6.84	1.8	254	0	18	0	0.18	216
rutabagas, ckd, bld, drnd, wo/salt	1 cup, cubes	30	0.93	0.18	6.84	1.8	5	0	18	0	0.18	216
rutabagas, raw	1 cup, cubes	37	1.08	0.16	8.62	2.3	12	0	43	0	0.44	305
rye flour, dark	1 cup	325	15.91	2.22	68.63	23.8	2	0	37	0	4.97	717
rye flour, light	1 cup	357	9.82	1.33	76.68	8	2	0	13	0	0.91	224

225

Food	Serving	Cals	Protein (g)	Fat (g)	Carbs (g)	Fiber (g)	Sodium (mg)	Cholesterol (mg)	Calcium (mg)	Vit D (IU)	Iron (mg)	Potassium (mg)
rye flour, medium	1 cup	349	10.88	1.52	75.43	11.8	2	0	24	0	2.54	374
rye grain	1 cup	338	10.34	1.63	75.86	15.1	2	0	24	0	2.63	510
saffron	1 tsp	310	11.43	5.85	65.37	3.9	148	0	111	0	11.1	1724
sage, ground	1 tsp	315	10.63	12.75	60.73	40.3	11	0	1652	0	28.12	1070
salad dressing, coleslaw	1 tbsp	390	0.9	33.4	23.8	0.1	710	26	14	3	0.2	9
salad drsng, bacon&tomato	1 tbsp	326	1.8	35	2	0.2	905	4	4	0	0.27	108
salad drsng, blue or roquefort chs drsng, comm, reg	1 tbsp	484	1.37	51.1	4.77	0.4	642	31	37	3	0.09	88
salad drsng, blue or roquefort chs, lo cal	1 tbsp	99	5.1	7.2	2.9	0	939	1	89	0	0.5	5
salad drsng, bttrmlk, lite	1 tablespoon	202	1.25	12.42	21.33	1.1	1120	16	40	0	0.69	132
salad drsng, caesar drsng, reg	1 tbsp	542	2.17	57.85	3.3	0.5	1209	39	48	5	1.08	29
salad drsng, caesar, fat-free	2 tbsp	131	1.47	0.23	30.73	0.2	1265	1	33	0	0.29	48
salad drsng, caesar, lo cal	1 tbsp	110	0.3	4.4	18.6	0.1	1148	2	24	0	0.18	29
salad drsng, coleslaw drsng, red fat	1 tbsp	329	0	20	40	0.4	1600	25	36	0	0.26	50
salad drsng, french drsng, comm, reg	1 tbsp	457	0.77	44.81	15.58	0	836	0	24	0	0.8	67
salad drsng, grn goddess, reg	1 tbsp	427	1.9	43.33	7.36	0	867	40	34	0	0.35	58
salad drsng, home recipe, vinegar&oil	1 tablespoon	449	0	50.1	2.5	0	1	0	0	0	0	8
salad drsng, honey mustard, reg	2 tbsp	464	0.87	40.83	23.33	0.4	512	29	12	6	0.29	20
salad drsng, italian drsng, comm, red fat	1 tablespoon	102	0.39	6.68	9.99	0	891	0	15	0	0.25	90
salad drsng, italian drsng, comm, reg	1 tbsp	240	0.41	21.12	12.12	0	993	0	13	0	0.26	84
salad drsng, mayo & mayonnaise-type, lo cal	1 tbsp	263	0.9	19	23.9	0	837	26	14	0	0.26	24
salad drsng, mayo type, reg, w/salt	1 tbsp	250	0.65	21.6	14.78	0	653	19	5	0	0.12	36
salad drsng, mayo, imitn, milk crm	1 tablespoon	97	2.1	5.1	11.1	0	504	43	72		0.5	97
salad drsng, mayo, imitn, soybn	1 tbsp	232	0.3	19.2	16	0	497	24	0	0	0	10
salad drsng, mayo, imitn, soybn wo/chol	1 tablespoon	482	0.1	47.7	15.8	0	353	0	0	0	0.01	10
salad drsng, mayo, lt	1 tablespoon	238	0.37	22.22	9.23	0	827	16	6	0	0.14	31
salad drsng, mayo, lt, smart balance, omega plus lt	1 tbsp	333	1.53	34.18	9.39	0.2	848	33	13		0.31	63
salad drsng, mayo, reg	1 tablespoon	680	0.96	74.85	0.57	0	635	42	8	7	0.21	20
salad drsng, mayo, soybn oil, wo/salt	1 tablespoon	717	1.1	79.4	2.7	0	30	59	18		0.5	34
salad drsng, mayo, soybn&safflower oil, w/salt	1 tablespoon	717	1.1	79.4	2.7	0	568	59	18		0.5	34
salad drsng, mayonnaise-like, fat-free	1 tbsp	84	0.2	2.7	15.5	1.9	788	9	6	0	0.12	49
salad drsng, mayonnaise-type, lt	1 tbsp	158	0.65	10	16.4	0	833	0	5	0	0.12	36
salad drsng, peppercorn drsng, comm, reg	1 tbsp	564	1.2	61.4	3.5	0	1103	49	22	4	0.35	176
salad drsng, poppyseed, creamy	2 tbsp	399	0.92	33.33	23.73	0.3	933	15	59	4	0.25	61
salad drsng, ranch drsng, fat-free	1 tablespoon	119	0.25	1.92	26.51	0.1	897	7	50		1.05	111
salad drsng, ranch drsng, red fat	1 tablespoon	196	1.25	12.42	21.33	1.1	1120	16	40	0	0.69	132
salad drsng, ranch drsng, reg	1 tablespoon	430	1.32	44.54	5.9	0	901	26	28	3	0.3	64
salad drsng, russian drsng	1 tbsp	355	0.69	26.18	31.9	0.7	1133	0	13	0	0.6	173
salad drsng, russian drsng, lo cal	1 tablespoon	141	0.5	4	27.6	0.3	868	6	19	0	0.6	157
salad drsng, sesame sd drsng, reg	1 tablespoon	443	3.1	45.2	8.6	1	1000	0	19	0	0.6	157
salad drsng, spray-style drsng, assorted flavors	10 sprays	165	0.16	10.75	16.6	0.3	1102	0	6		0.18	
salad drsng, swt&sour	1 tbsp	15	0.1	0	3.7	0	208	0	4	0	0.04	33
salami ckd bf	1 slice	261	12.6	22.2	1.9	0	1140	71	6	48	2.2	188
salami italian pork	1 oz	425	21.7	37	1.2	0	1890	80	10		1.52	340
salami italian pork & bf dry sliced 50% less na	1 serving, 5 slices	350	21.8	26.4	6.4	0	936	89	8		1.51	378
salami pork bf less na	3.527 oz	396	15.01	30.5	15.38	0.2	623	90	94	32	1.55	1372
salami, ckd, bf&pork	1 slice, round	336	21.85	25.9	2.4	0	1740	89	15	41	1.56	316
salami, cooked, turkey	1 serving	172	19.2	9.21	1.55	0.1	1107	76	40	24	1.25	216
salami, dry or hard, pork	1 package, (4 oz)	407	22.58	33.72	1.6	0	2260	79	13		1.3	378
salami, dry or hard, pork, bf	1 slice	378	21.07	31.65	0.72	0	1756	108	24	36	1.36	363
salisbury steak w/ gravy, frz	1 patty	149	6.98	10.47	6.78	1	509	33	47	1	0.95	144
salmon, atlantic, farmed, ckd, dry heat	3 oz	206	22.1	12.35	0	0	61	63	15	526	0.34	384
salmon, atlantic, wild, ckd, dry heat	3 oz	182	25.44	8.13	0	0	56	71	15		1.03	628
salmon, chinook, ckd, dry heat	3 oz	231	25.72	13.38	0	0	60	85	28		0.91	505

Food	Serving	Cals	Protein (g)	Fat (g)	Carbs (g)	Fiber (g)	Sodium (mg)	Cholesterol (mg)	Calcium (mg)	Vit D (IU)	Iron (mg)	Potassium (mg)
salmon, chinook, smoked	1 oz, boneless	117	18.28	4.32	0	0	672	23	11	685	0.85	175
salmon, chinook, smoked, (lox), reg	1 oz	117	18.28	4.32	0	0	2000	23	11		0.85	175
salmon, chum, ckd, dry heat	3 oz	154	25.82	4.83	0	0	64	95	14		0.71	550
salmon, chum, cnd, wo/salt, drnd sol w/bone	3 oz	141	21.43	5.5	0	0	75	39	249		0.7	300
salmon, chum, drnd sol w/bone	3 oz	141	21.43	5.5	0	0	391	39	249	386	0.7	300
salmon, coho, farmed, ckd, dry heat	1 fillet	178	24.3	8.23	0	0	52	63	12		0.39	460
salmon, coho, wild, ckd, dry heat	3 oz	139	23.45	4.3	0	0	58	55	45	451	0.61	434
salmon, coho, wild, ckd, moist heat	3 oz	184	27.36	7.5	0	0	53	57	46		0.71	455
salmon, pink, ckd, dry heat	3 oz	153	24.58	5.28	0	0	90	55	8	522	0.45	439
salmon, pink, cnd, drnd sol, wo/ skn & bones	3 oz	136	24.62	4.21	0	0	378	83	60	563	0.57	326
salmon, pink, cnd, wo/salt, sol w/ bone&liq	3 oz	139	19.78	6.05	0	0	75	55	213		0.84	326
salmon, red (sockeye), filets w/ skn, smoked (alaska native)	1 filet	345	60.62	11.43	0	0	51	155	58		1.06	960
salmon, sockeye, ckd, dry heat	3 oz	156	26.48	5.57	0	0	92	61	11	670	0.52	436
salmon, sockeye, cnd, drnd sol, wo/ skn & bones	3 oz	158	26.33	5.87	0	0	386	66	37	859	0.48	312
salmon, sockeye, cnd, total can contents	3 oz	153	20.63	7.17	0	0	433	67	198	761	0.57	329
salmon, sockeye, cnd, wo/salt, drnd sol w/bone	3 oz	153	20.47	7.31	0	0	75	44	239		1.06	377
salsify, ckd, bld, drnd, w/salt	1 cup, slices	68	2.73	0.17	15.36	3.1	252	0	47	0	0.55	283
salsify, ckd, bld, drnd, wo/salt	1 cup, sliced	68	2.73	0.17	15.36	3.1	16	0	47	0	0.55	283
salt, table	1 tsp	0	0	0	0	0	38758	0	24	0	0.33	8
sardine, atlantic, cnd in oil, drnd sol w/bone	1 cup, drained	208	24.62	11.45	0	0	307	142	382	193	2.92	397
sardine, pacific, cnd in tomato sau, drnd sol w/bone	1 cup	185	20.86	10.45	0.54	0.1	414	61	240	193	2.3	341
sauce, alfredo mix, dry	.25 cup	535	15.32	36.35	36.52	2	2590	56	467		0.94	254
sauce, barbecue	1 tbsp	172	0.82	0.63	40.77	0.9	1027	0	33	0	0.64	232
sauce, chs sau mix, dry	.25 cup	438	7.68	18.33	60.52	1	3202	23	204		0.5	428
sauce, chs, rts	.25 cup	174	6.71	13.29	6.83	0.5	828	29	184		0.21	30
sauce, cocktail, rts	.25 cup	124	1.36	1.05	28.22	1.8	983	0	26	0	0.83	309
sauce, duck, rts	2 tbsp	245	0.36	0.13	60.61	0.6	455	0	11	0	0.39	87
sauce, enchilada, red, mild, ready to serve	.25 cup	30	0.62	0.91	4.87	0.5	547	0	7	0	0.67	101
sauce, hoisin, rts	1 tbsp	220	3.31	3.39	44.08	2.8	1615	3	32	0	1.01	119
sauce, homemade, white, med	1 cup	147	3.84	10.63	9.17	0.2	354	7	118	48	0.33	156
sauce, homemade, white, thick	1 cup	186	3.99	13.83	11.61	0.3	373	6	111	47	0.5	149
sauce, homemade, white, thin	1 cup	105	3.77	6.73	7.4	0.1	328	8	126	49	0.21	163
sauce, horseradish	1 tsp	503	1.09	50.89	10.05	1	730	50	12	10	0.23	44
sauce, hot chile, sriracha	1 tsp	93	1.93	0.93	19.16	2.2	2124		18		1.64	321
sauce, hot chile, sriracha, cha! by texas pete	1 tsp	108	2.02	0.98	22.73	2.1	2903		15		1.46	302
sauce, hot chile, sriracha, tuong ot sriracha	1 tsp	79	1.86	0.9	15.87	2.2	1540		20		1.92	341
sauce, old el paso, enchilada, red, mild, ready to serve	.25 cup	29	0.59	0.67	5.04	0.6	543		6		0.29	97
sauce, oyster, rts	1 tbsp	51	1.35	0.25	10.92	0.3	2733	0	32	0	0.18	54
sauce, pasta, spaghetti/marinara, rts	.5 cup	50	1.39	1.61	7.43	1.8	437	2	26	0	0.73	320
sauce, pasta, spaghetti/marinara, rts, lo na	.5 cup	51	1.41	1.48	8.06	1.8	30	2	27	0	0.78	319
sauce, peppers, hot, chili, mature red, cnd	1 tbsp	21	0.9	0.6	3.9	0.7	25	0	9	0	0.5	564
sauce, pesto, rts, refr	.25 cup	418	9.83	37.6	10.09	1.8	603		306		0.57	560
sauce, pesto, rts, shelf stable	.25 cup	426	5	42.42	6.14	1.7	998		173		0.88	205
sauce, pizza, cnd, rts	.25 cup	54	2.18	1.15	8.66	2	348	0	54		0.9	354
sauce, plum, ready-to-serve	1 tbsp	184	0.89	1.04	42.81	0.7	538	0	12		1.43	259
sauce, pnut, made from cocnt, h2o, sugar, pnuts	1 tbsp	179	2.02	6.34	28.46	1.1	319	0	9	0	0.38	99

Food	Serving	Cals	Protein (g)	Fat (g)	Carbs (g)	Fiber (g)	Sodium (mg)	Cholesterol (mg)	Calcium (mg)	Vit D (IU)	Iron (mg)	Potassium (mg)
sauce, pnut, made from pnut butter, h2o, soy sau	1 tbsp	257	6.31	16.02	22.02	1.8	1338	0	22	0	0.91	235
sauce, ready-to-serve	1 tbsp	35	5.06	0.01	3.64	0	7851	0	43	0	0.78	288
sauce, rts, pepper or hot	1 tsp	11	0.51	0.37	1.75	0.3	2643	0	8		0.48	144
sauce, rts, pepper, tabasco	1 tsp	12	1.29	0.76	0.8	0.6	633	0	12	0	1.16	128
sauce, salsa, rts	2 tbsp	29	1.52	0.17	6.64	1.9	711	0	30	0	0.42	275
sauce, salsa, verde, rts	2 tbsp	38	1.13	0.89	6.36	1.9	600	0	9	0	0.65	259
sauce, sofrito, prep from recipe	.5 cup	237	12.8	18.2	5.46	1.7	1145		20		0.94	401
sauce, steak, tomato bsd	2 tbsp	95	1.25	0.23	22.04	1.5	1647	0	19	0	1.37	312
sauce, swt & sour, prepared-from-recipe	2 tbsp	79	1.84	0.58	16.72	0.4	347	1	16		0.67	193
sauce, swt & sour, rts	2 tbsp	150	0.27	0.02	38.22	0.1	371	0	10	0	0.21	99
sauce, tartar, rts	2 tablespoons	211	1	16.7	13.3	0.5	667	7	26	2	0.25	68
sauce, teriyaki, rts	1 tbsp	89	5.93	0.02	15.56	0.1	3833	0	25	0	1.7	225
sauce, teriyaki, rts, red na	2 tbsp	89	5.93	0.02	15.58	0.1	1778	0	25	0	1.7	225
sauce, tomato chili sau, btld, w/salt	1 packet	92	2.5	0.3	19.79	2.4	1338	0	20	0	0.8	370
sauce, white, thin, prepared-from-recipe, w/ butter	1 tbsp	72	3.95	2.56	8.29	0.1	184	8	131		0.22	167
sauce, worcestershire	1 tbsp	78	0	0	19.46	0	980	0	107	0	5.3	800
sauerkraut, cnd, sol&liquids	1 cup	19	0.91	0.14	4.28	2.9	661	0	30	0	1.47	170
sausage berliner pork bf	1 slice	230	15.27	17.2	2.59	0	1297	46	12	13	1.15	283
sausage chick bf pork skinless smoked	1 link	216	13.6	14.3	8.1	0	1034	120	100		4.8	246
sausage italian swt links	3 oz	149	16.13	8.42	2.1	0	570	30	25		1.19	194
sausage italian turkey smoked	2 oz	158	15.05	8.75	4.65	0.9	928	53	21		9.6	197
sausage polish bf w/ chick hot	5 pieces	259	17.6	19.4	3.6	0	1540	66	12		0.88	237
sausage polish pork & bf smoked	2.67 oz	301	12.07	26.56	1.98	0	848	71	7	44	1	189
sausage pork & bf w/ cheddar chs smoked	12 oz	296	12.89	25.84	2.13	0	848	63	57	12	0.73	206
sausage smmr pork & bf stks w/ cheddar chs	1 oz	426	19.43	37.91	1.82	0.2	1483	89	81	12	2.26	206
sausage turkey brkfst links mild	2 oz, 2 links	235	15.42	18.09	1.56	0	639	160	32	17	1.07	229
sausage turkey hot smoked	2 oz	158	15.05	8.75	4.65	0.3	916	53	21	8	9.6	197
sausage, chick or turkey, italian style, lower na	2 oz	183	21.43	4.46	14.25	0	446	36	0	5	1.29	1062
sausage, egg & chs brkfst biscuit	1 biscuit	324	9.54	22.13	21.57	2	591	78	136	27	1.85	269
sausage, italian, pork, ckd	1 link	344	19.12	27.31	4.27	0.1	743	57	21	41	1.43	304
sausage, italian, pork, raw	1 link	346	14.25	31.33	0.65	0	731	76	18		1.18	253
sausage, meatless	1 link	255	20.28	18.16	8.09	2.8	888	0	63	0	3.72	231
sausage, pork, turkey, & bf, red na	3 oz	284	10.71	26.79	0.11	0.1	679	70	24	3	1.6	240
sausage, smoked link sausage, pork & bf	3 oz	320	12	28.73	2.42	0	911	58	12	44	0.75	179
sausage, vienna, cnd, chick, bf, pork	1 sausage	230	10.5	19.4	2.6	0	879	87	10	25	0.88	101
savory, ground	1 tsp	272	6.73	5.91	68.73	45.7	24	0	2132	0	37.88	1051
scallop, (bay&sea), ckd, stmd	3 oz	111	20.54	0.84	5.41	0	667	41	10	2	0.58	314
scallop, mixed species, raw	5 small scallops	69	12.06	0.49	3.18	0	392	24	6	1	0.38	205
scallop, mxd sp, ckd, breaded&fried	2 large	216	18.07	10.94	10.13		464	54	42		0.82	333
scallop, mxd sp, imitn, made from surimi	3 oz	99	12.77	0.41	10.62	0	795	22	8		0.31	103
sea bass, mxd sp, ckd, dry heat	1 fillet	124	23.63	2.56	0	0	87	53	13		0.37	328
seasoning mix, dry, chili, original	1.33 tbsp	335	10.82	7.3	56.56	10.8	4616	0	0		3.9	
seasoning mix, dry, sazon, coriander & annatto	.25 tsp	0	0	0	0	0	17000	0	0		0	
seasoning mix, dry, taco, original	2 tsp	322	4.5	0	58	13.3	7203	0	0		7.2	1000
seatrout, mxd sp, ckd, dry heat	3 oz	133	21.46	4.63	0	0	74	106	24		0.35	437
seaweed, agar, dried	.25 cup	306	6.21	0.3	80.88	7.7	102	0	625	0	21.4	1125
seaweed, canadian cultivated emi-tsunomata, dry	.25 cup	259	15.34	1.39	46.24	36.7	4331	33	299	126	66.38	2944
seaweed, canadian cultivated emi-tsunomata, rehydrated	.25 cup	31	1.86	0.17	5.62	4.5	526		36	15	8.07	358
seaweed, spirulina, dried	1 cup	290	57.47	7.72	23.9	3.6	1048	0	120	0	28.5	1363
semisweet choc	1 serving	480	4.2	30	63.9	5.9	11	0	32	0	3.13	365
semisweet choc, made w/butter	1 cup, chips	477	4.2	29.7	63.4	5.9	11	18	32		3.13	365
sesame crunch	1 oz	516	11.6	33.3	50.3	7.7	167	0	639	0	4.27	307

Food	Serving	Cals	Protein (g)	Fat (g)	Carbs (g)	Fiber (g)	Sodium (mg)	Cholesterol (mg)	Calcium (mg)	Vit D (IU)	Iron (mg)	Potassium (mg)
sesame whl, rstd&tstd	1 oz	565	16.96	48	25.74	14	11	0	989	0	14.76	475
sesame whole, dried	1 cup	573	17.73	49.67	23.45	11.8	11	0	975	0	14.55	468
shake, strawberry	1 fl oz	113	3.4	2.8	18.9	0.4	83	11	113	0	0.11	182
shallots, freeze-dried	1 tbsp	348	12.3	0.5	80.7	15.7	59	0	183	0	6	1650
shallots, raw	1 tbsp, chopped	72	2.5	0.1	16.8	3.2	12	0	37	0	1.2	334
sherbet, orange	.5 cup	144	1.1	2	30.4	1.3	46	1	54	0	0.14	96
shortening bread, soybn (hydr)&cttnsd	1 tablespoon	884	0	100	0	0	0	0	0		0	0
shortening cake mix, soybn (hydr)&cttnsd (hydr)	1 tbsp	884	0	100	0	0	0	0	0	0	0	0
shortening confectionery, cocnt (hydr)&or palm kernel (hydr)	1 tbsp	884	0	100	0	0	0	0	0	0	0	0
shortening frying (hvy duty), bf tallow&cttnsd	1 tbsp	900	0	100	0	0	0	100	0		0	0
shortening frying (hvy duty), palm (hydr)	1 tbsp	884	0	100	0	0	0	0	0		0	0
shortening frying hvy duty, soybn hydr, linoleic (less than 1%)	1 tbsp	884	0	100	0	0	0	0	0		0	0
shortening household soybn (hydr)&palm	1 tbsp	884	0	100	0	0	0	0	0		0	0
shortening, household, lard&veg oil	1 tablespoon	900	0	100	0	0	0	56	0	0	0	0
shortening, veg, household, comp	1 tbsp	884	0	99.97	0	0	4	0	1	0	0.07	0
shrimp, breaded&fried	3 pieces, shrimp	308	7.84	18.9	27.99	0.7	897	58	29	1	0.86	82
shrimp, mxd sp, ckd, breaded&fried	3 oz	242	21.39	12.28	11.47	0.4	344	138	67	5	1.26	225
shrimp, mxd sp, cnd	1 cup	100	20.42	1.36	0	0	870	252	145	0	2.13	80
shrimp, mxd sp, imitn, made from surimi	3 oz	101	12.39	1.47	9.13	0	705	36	19		0.6	89
smoked link sausage, pork	1 link	309	11.98	28.23	0.94	0	827	61	11	43	0.59	483
smoked link sausage, pork&bf, nonfat dry milk	1 link	313	13.28	27.61	1.92	0	1173	65	41		1.47	286
snapper, mxd sp, ckd, dry heat	3 oz	128	26.3	1.72	0	0	57	47	40		0.24	522
soda, orange	1 fl oz	48	0	0	12.3	0	12	0	5		0.06	2
soda, other than cola or pepper, wo/ caffeine, lo cal	1 fl oz	0	0.1	0	0	0	6	0	4	0	0.04	2
soft fruit & nut squares	3 pieces	390	2.31	9.52	73.81	2.4	131	0	17	0	0.93	82
soup, bean w/ frankfurters, cnd, cond	1 cup	142	7.6	5.31	16.75	4.6	831	9	66		1.78	363
soup, bean w/ frankfurters, cnd, prep w/ eq volume h2o	1 cup	75	3.99	2.79	8.8		437	5	35		0.94	191
soup, bean w/ ham, cnd, chunky, rts	1 cup	95	5.19	3.5	11.16	4.6	400	9	32		1.33	175
soup, bean w/ pork, cnd, cond	.5 cup	129	5.88	4.42	16.97	5.9	672	2	60	0	1.53	375
soup, bean w/ pork, cnd, prep w/ eq volume h2o	1 cup	63	2.88	2.16	8.31	2.9	349	1	31	0	0.75	147
soup, bean w/bacon, cond, single brand	.5 cup	117	6.5	2.1	18	4.6	672	3			1.37	
soup, bean&ham, cnd, red na, prep w/h2o or rts	1 cup	81	4.19	1.03	13.66	4	187	2	38	0	1.02	158
soup, beef broth, cubed, dry	1 cube	170	17.3	4	16.1	0	24000	4	60	0	2.23	403
soup, bf & mushroom, lo na, chunk style	1 cup	69	4.3	2.3	9.58	0.2	25	6	13	0	0.97	140
soup, bf & veg, cnd, rts	1 cup	48	3.18	1.16	6.16	1.2	326	7	18	1	0.51	174
soup, bf & veg, red na, cnd, rts	1 cup	42	3.26	0.95	4.99	0.8	175		17		0.45	277
soup, bf barley, ready to serve	1 cup	52	2.81	0.96	7.94	0.9	297	4	11	0	0.45	121
soup, bf broth bouillon & consomme, cnd, cond	.5 cup	11	2.52	0	0.32	0	694	0	7		0.43	125
soup, bf broth or bouillon cnd, rts	1 cup	7	1.14	0.22	0.04	0	372	0	6	0	0.17	54
soup, bf broth or bouillon, pdr, dry	1 cube	213	15.97	8.89	17.4	0	26000	10	60	0	1	446
soup, bf broth or bouillon, pdr, prep w/h2o	1 cup	3	0.21	0.08	0.25	0	382	0	4	0	0.02	6
soup, bf broth, bouillon, consomme, prep w/ eq volume h2o	1 cup	12	2.22	0	0.73	0	264	0	4		0.22	64
soup, bf broth, cubed, prep w/h2o	1 cup	3	0.21	0.08	0.25	0	260	0	4	0	0.02	6
soup, bf broth, less/reduced na, ready to serve	1 cup	6	1.14	0.07	0.2	0	225	0	3	0	0.04	20
soup, bf mushroom, cnd, cond	.5 cup	61	4.6	2.4	5.2	0.2	709	5	4		0.7	126

Food	Serving	Cals	Protein (g)	Fat (g)	Carbs (g)	Fiber (g)	Sodium (mg)	Cholesterol (mg)	Calcium (mg)	Vit D (IU)	Iron (mg)	Potassium (mg)
soup, bf mushroom, cnd, prep w/ eq volume h2o	1 cup	30	2.37	1.23	2.6	0.1	386	3	2		0.36	63
soup, bf noodle, cnd, cond	.5 cup	67	3.85	2.46	7.16	0.6	653	4	12	0	0.88	79
soup, bf noodle, cnd, prep w/ eq volume h2o	1 cup	34	1.93	1.23	3.58	0.3	325	2	8	0	0.44	40
soup, bf stroganoff, cnd, chunky style, rts	1 cup	98	5.1	4.6	9	0.6	435	21	20	0	0.88	140
soup, bf w/veg&barley, cnd, cond, single brand	1 serving	61	3.9	1.4	8.2		707	6				
soup, black bean, cnd, cond	1 cup	91	4.83	1.32	15.42	6.8	970	0	35		1.5	250
soup, black bean, cnd, prep w/ eq volume h2o	1 cup	46	2.42	0.66	7.71	3.4	487	0	19	0	0.75	125
soup, bouillon cubes&granules, lo na, dry	1 tsp	438	16.7	13.89	64.88	0.2	1067	13	187	0	1.03	309
soup, broccoli chs, cnd, cond, comm	1/2 cup	87	2.1	5.3	7.7	1.8	661	4	41	0	0.3	207
soup, chick & veg, cnd, rts	1 cup	33	1.97	0.73	4.68	0.9	229	3	14	0	0.25	133
soup, chick broth cubes, dry	1 cube	198	14.6	4.7	23.5	0	24000	13	190		1.87	374
soup, chick broth cubes, dry, prep w/ h2o	1 cup	5	0.39	0.12	0.62		326	0	5		0.05	10
soup, chick broth or bouillon, dry	1 cube	267	16.66	13.88	18.01	0	23875	13	187	0	1.03	309
soup, chick broth or bouillon, dry, prep w/ h2o	1 cup	4	0.28	0.23	0.3	0	401	0	6	0	0.02	6
soup, chick broth, cnd, cond	.5 cup	31	4.42	1.04	0.75	0	621	1	6	0	0.41	170
soup, chick broth, cnd, prep w/ eq volume h2o	1 cup	16	2.02	0.57	0.38	0	306	0	4	0	0.21	86
soup, chick broth, less/reduced na, ready to serve	1 cup	7	1.36	0	0.38	0	231	0	8	0	0.26	85
soup, chick broth, lo na, cnd	1 cup	16	2	0.6	1.2	0	30	0	4	0	0.21	86
soup, chick broth, rts	1 cup	6	0.64	0.21	0.44	0	371	2	4	0	0.07	18
soup, chick corn chowder, chunky, rts, single brand	1 serving	99	3.1	6.3	7.5	0.9	299	11				
soup, chick gumbo, cnd, cond	.5 cup	45	2.1	1.14	6.67	1.6	693	3	19		0.71	60
soup, chick gumbo, cnd, prep w/ eq volume h2o	1 cup	23	1.08	0.59	3.43	0.8	391	2	10	0	0.37	31
soup, chick mushroom chowder, chunky, rts, single brand	1 serving	80	3	4.4	7.1	1.4	339	6			0.48	
soup, chick mushroom, cnd, cond	.5 cup	100	1.61	4.84	11.95	3.2	669	8	23	0	0.7	56
soup, chick mushroom, cnd, prep w/ eq volume h2o	1 cup	54	1.8	3.75	3.8	0.1	327	4	12		0.36	63
soup, chick noodle, cnd, cond	.5 cup	48	2.37	1.55	6.07	0.9	681	8	6	0	0.67	48
soup, chick noodle, cnd, prep w/ eq volume h2o	1 cup	24	1.16	0.76	2.97	0.5	335	4	5	0	0.33	24
soup, chick noodle, dry, mix	1 packet	377	15.42	6.51	62.32	3.2	3643	74	55	0	2.44	306
soup, chick noodle, dry, mix, prep w/ h2o	1 cup	23	0.84	0.55	3.67	0.1	229	4	2	0	0.2	13
soup, chick noodle, lo na, cnd, prep w/ eq volume h2o	1 cup	25	1.27	0.95	2.95	0.2	173	5	6	0	0.66	22
soup, chick noodle, red na, cnd, rts	1 cup	41	3.29	1.34	3.84	0.8	186	4	11	0	0.33	285
soup, chick rice, cnd, chunky, rts	1 cup	53	5.11	1.33	5.41	0.4	370	5	14	0	0.78	45
soup, chick veg w/potato&chs, chunky, rts	1 cup	65	1.16	4.46	5.2	0.3	416	7	15	0	0.16	73
soup, chick veg, chunky, red fat, red na, rts, single brand	1 serving	40	2.7	0.5	6.3		192	4				
soup, chick veg, cnd, cond	.5 cup	61	2.94	2.32	7.01	0.7	706	7	14	0	0.71	126
soup, chick w/ rice, cnd, cond	.5 cup	68	1.84	1.56	11.57	0.9	645	4	41	0	0.25	34
soup, chick w/ rice, cnd, prep w/ eq volume h2o	1 cup	24	1.45	0.78	2.92	0.3	238	3	9	0	0.31	41
soup, chick w/star-shaped pasta, cnd, cond, single brand	1 serving	50	2.3	1.4	7.1		732	4				
soup, chick, cnd, chunky, rts	1 cup	71	5.06	2.64	6.88	0.6	354	12	10	0	0.69	70
soup, chili bf, cnd, cond	1 cup	117	5.09	2.53	18.86	2.5	788	10	33		1.62	400
soup, chili bf, cnd, prep w/ eq volume h2o	1 cup	57	2.49	1.24	9.23	1.2	388	5	18	0	0.79	196
soup, chs, cnd, cond	.5 cup	82	0.8	3.92	11.3	2.2	692	3	36	0	0.15	37
soup, chs, cnd, prep w/ eq volume h2o	1 cup	63	2.19	4.24	4.26	0.4	388	12	57		0.3	62

Food	Serving	Cals	Protein (g)	Fat (g)	Carbs (g)	Fiber (g)	Sodium (mg)	Cholesterol (mg)	Calcium (mg)	Vit D (IU)	Iron (mg)	Potassium (mg)
soup, chs, cnd, prep w/ eq volume milk	1 cup	92	3.77	5.8	6.47	0.4	406	19	115		0.32	136
soup, clam chowder, manhattan style, cnd, chunky, rts	1 cup	56	3.02	1.41	7.84	1.2	417	6	28	0	1.1	160
soup, clam chowder, manhattan, cnd, cond	.5 cup	61	1.74	1.76	9.74	1.2	698	2	19		1.3	150
soup, clam chowder, manhattan, cnd, prep w/eq volume h2o	1 cup	30	0.85	0.86	4.77	0.6	226	1	11	0	0.64	74
soup, clam chowder, new eng, cnd, prep w/ eq vlm lofat (2%) milk	1 cup	61	3.24	2.02	7.46	0.3	273	7	70	25	1.21	179
soup, crm of asparagus, cnd, cond	.5 cup	69	1.82	3.26	8.52	0.4	669	4	23	0	0.64	138
soup, crm of asparagus, cnd, prep w/ eq volume h2o	1 cup	35	0.94	1.68	4.38	0.2	402	2	12		0.33	71
soup, crm of asparagus, cnd, prep w/ eq volume milk	1 cup	65	2.55	3.3	6.61	0.3	420	9	70		0.35	145
soup, crm of celery, cnd, cond	.5 cup	72	1.32	4.46	7.03	0.6	516	11	32	0	0.5	98
soup, crm of celery, cnd, prep w/ eq volume h2o	1 cup	37	0.68	2.29	3.62	0.3	254	6	16		0.26	50
soup, crm of celery, cnd, prep w/ eq volume milk	1 cup	66	2.29	3.91	5.86	0.3	272	13	75		0.28	125
soup, crm of chick, cnd, cond	.5 cup	90	2.38	5.77	7.16	0	702	8	14	0	1.06	49
soup, crm of chick, cnd, cond, red na	.5 cup	58	1.8	1.3	9.5	0.4	357	6	11	0	0.2	272
soup, crm of chick, cnd, cond, single brand	1 serving	99	2.4	6.5	7.7		788	7				
soup, crm of chick, cnd, prep w/ eq volume h2o	1 cup	48	1.41	3.02	3.8	0.1	347	4	14		0.25	36
soup, crm of chick, cnd, prep w/ eq volume milk	1 cup	77	3.01	4.62	6.04	0.1	362	11	73		0.27	110
soup, crm of chick, dry, mix, prep w/ h2o	1 cup	41	0.68	2.04	5.11	0.1	454	1	29	0	0.1	82
soup, crm of mushroom, cnd, cond	.5 cup	79	1.35	5.3	6.8	0.7	691	0	12	9	0.18	64
soup, crm of mushroom, cnd, cond, red na	1 cup	52	1.21	1.69	8.1	0.6	383	3	13	0	0.48	374
soup, crm of mushroom, cnd, prep w/ eq volume h2o	1 cup	39	0.66	2.59	3.33	0.3	340	0	7	4	0.09	31
soup, crm of mushroom, cnd, prep w/ eq volume lofat (2%) milk	1 cup	65	2.36	3.58	5.76	0.3	357	4	68	29	0.1	103
soup, crm of mushroom, lo na, rts, cnd	1 cup	53	1	3.7	4.53	0.2	20	1	19	0	0.21	41
soup, crm of onion, cnd, cond	.5 cup	88	2.2	4.2	10.4	0.4	637	12	27	0	0.5	98
soup, crm of onion, cnd, prep w/ eq volume h2o	1 cup	44	1.13	2.16	5.2	0.4	380	6	14		0.26	49
soup, crm of onion, cnd, prep w/ eq volume milk	1 cup	75	2.74	3.78	7.4	0.3	405	13	72		0.28	125
soup, crm of potato, cnd, cond	.5 cup	74	1.51	1.88	12.79	1.3	604	1	17	0	0.34	165
soup, crm of potato, cnd, prep w/ eq volume h2o	1 cup	30	0.72	0.97	4.7	0.2	238	2	8		0.2	56
soup, crm of potato, cnd, prep w/ eq volume milk	1 cup	60	2.33	2.6	6.92	0.2	230	9	67		0.22	130
soup, crm of shrimp, cnd, cond	.5 cup	72	2.22	4.14	6.53	0.2	685	13	14		0.42	47
soup, crm of shrimp, cnd, prep w/ eq volume h2o	1 cup	36	1.11	2.07	3.27	0.1	391	7	9	0	0.21	24
soup, crm of shrimp, cnd, prep w/ eq volume lofat (2%) milk	1 cup	61	2.78	3.23	5.64	0.1	354	10	69	25	0.22	95
soup, crm of veg, dry, pdr	1 packet	446	8	24.1	52.1	3	4957	2	134	0	2.6	408
soup, egg drop, chinese restaurant	1 cup	27	1.16	0.61	4.29	0.4	370	23	7	6	0.26	22
soup, homemade (alaska native)	1 cup	72	7.4	2.2	5.6		30	12	35		0.5	128
soup, hot & sour, chinese restaurant	1 cup	39	2.58	1.21	4.35	0.5	376	21	19	5	0.64	55
soup, lentil w/ham, cnd, rts	1 cup	56	3.74	1.12	8.16		532	3	17		1.07	144
soup, minestrone, cnd, chunky, rts	1 cup	53	2.13	1.17	8.64	2.4	288	2	25	0	0.74	255
soup, minestrone, cnd, cond	.5 cup	68	3.48	2.05	9.17	0.8	516	1	28	0	0.75	255
soup, minestrone, cnd, prep w/ eq volume h2o	1 cup	34	1.77	1.04	4.66	0.4	254	1	14		0.38	130
soup, minestrone, cnd, red na, rts	1 cup	50	2	0.8	9	2.4	215	0	20	0	0.72	186
soup, mushroom barley, cnd, cond	.5 cup	61	1.5	1.8	9.6		573	0	10		0.4	76
soup, mushroom barley, cnd, prep w/ eq volume h2o	1 cup	30	0.77	0.93	4.8	0.3	365	0	5		0.21	38

Food	Serving	Cals	Protein (g)	Fat (g)	Carbs (g)	Fiber (g)	Sodium (mg)	Cholesterol (mg)	Calcium (mg)	Vit D (IU)	Iron (mg)	Potassium (mg)
soup, mushroom w/ bf stock, cnd, cond	.5 cup	68	2.51	3.21	7.41	0.1	773	6	8	0	0.67	126
soup, mushroom w/ bf stock, cnd, prep w/ eq volume h2o	1 cup	35	1.29	1.65	3.81	0.3	397	3	4		0.34	65
soup, onion, cnd, cond	.5 cup	46	3.06	1.42	6.68	0.7	516	0	22	0	0.55	56
soup, onion, dry, mix	1 tbsp	293	7.48	0.34	65.07	6.6	8031	0	143	0	1.25	721
soup, onion, dry, mix, prep w/ h2o	1 cup	12	0.32	0.01	2.77	0.3	346	0	9	0	0.05	31
soup, oyster stew, cnd, cond	.5 cup	48	1.72	3.13	3.32	0	722	11	18		0.8	40
soup, oyster stew, cnd, prep w/ eq volume h2o	1 cup	24	0.87	1.59	1.69		407	6	9		0.41	20
soup, oyster stew, cnd, prep w/ eq volume milk	1 cup	55	2.51	3.24	3.99	0	425	13	68		0.43	96
soup, pea, grn, cnd, cond	.5 cup	125	6.54	2.23	20.18	3.9	680	0	21	0	1.48	145
soup, pea, grn, cnd, prep w/ eq volume h2o	1 cup	61	3.2	1.09	9.88	1.9	336	0	12	0	0.73	71
soup, pea, grn, cnd, prep w/ eq volume milk	1 cup	94	4.97	2.77	12.69	1.1	352	7	68		0.79	148
soup, pea, lo na, prep w/ eq volume h2o	1 cup	62	3.2	1.09	9.88	1.9	10	0	12	0	0.73	71
soup, pea, split w/ ham, cnd, cond	.5 cup	141	7.68	3.28	20.81	1.7	630	6	16		1.7	297
soup, pea, split w/ ham, cnd, prep w/ eq volume h2o	1 cup	75	4.08	1.74	11.05	0.9	398	3	9		0.9	158
soup, ramen noodle, any flavor, dry	1 package, without flavor packet	440	10.17	17.59	60.26	2.9	1855	0	21	0	4.11	181
soup, ramen noodle, bf flavor, dry	1 package, without flavor packet	441	10.06	17.73	60.34	3	1727		21		3.93	177
soup, ramen noodle, chick flavor, dry	1 package, without flavor packet	439	10.22	17.52	60.23	2.9	1923		22		4.21	183
soup, ramen noodle, dry, any flavor, red fat, red na	1.41 oz, dry (half noodle block)	350	10.89	2.5	70.95	2.7	1200	0	22	0	4.52	128
soup, sirloin burger w/veg, rts, single brand	1 cup	77	4.2	3.7	6.8	2.3	361	11			0.87	
soup, split pea w/ ham, chunky, red fat, red na, rts, single brand	1 cup	76	5.2	1.1	11.3		343	6			0.92	
soup, split pea w/ham&bacon, cnd, cond, single brand	1 cup	140	8.6	2.3	21.2	3	729	3			1.59	
soup, stock, beef, home-prepared	1 cup	13	1.97	0.09	1.2	0	198	0	8	0	0.27	185
soup, stock, chick, home-prepared	1 cup	36	2.52	1.2	3.53	0	143	3	3	0	0.21	105
soup, stock, home-prepared	1 cup	16	2.26	0.81	0	0	156	1	3	0	0.01	144
soup, tomato, cnd, prep w/ eq volume lofat (2%) milk	1 serving, 1 cup	55	2.42	1.24	9.82	0.5	206	4	68	25	0.3	343
soup, tomato, cnd, prep w/eq volume h2o, comm	1 cup	32	0.71	0.21	7.45	0.5	186	0	8	0	0.29	275
soup, tomato, dry, mix, prep w/ h2o	1 cup	38	0.93	0.61	7.17	0.4	356	2	29	0	0.18	111
soup, tomato, lo na, w/h2o	1 cup	30	0.79	0.28	6.57	0.6	33	0	8	0	0.54	112
soup, turkey noodle, cnd, prep w/ eq volume h2o	1 cup	28	1.6	0.82	3.54	0.3	334	2	5		0.39	31
soup, turkey veg, cnd, prep w/ eq volume h2o	1 cup	30	1.28	1.26	3.58	0.2	376	1	7		0.32	73
soup, turkey, chunky, cnd, rts	1 cup	57	4.33	1.87	5.96		391	4	21		0.81	153
soup, veg bf, cnd, cond	.5 cup	63	4.45	1.51	8.11	1.6	706	4	13	0	0.89	138
soup, veg bf, cnd, cond, single brand	1 serving	53	3.8	0.8	7.7		555	5				
soup, veg bf, cnd, prep w/ eq volume h2o	1 cup	31	2.23	0.76	4.06	0.8	349	2	8	0	0.45	69
soup, veg bf, microwavable, rts, single brand	1 serving	44	6.2	0.7	3.3	1.5	376	3				
soup, veg broth, ready to serve	1 cup	5	0.24	0.07	0.93	0	296	0	3	0	0.06	19
soup, veg chick, cnd, prep w/ h2o, lo na	1 cup	69	5.1	2	8.76	0.4	35	7	11	0	0.61	153
soup, veg soup, cond, lo na, prep w/ eq volume h2o	1 cup	33	1.1	0.45	6.06	1.1	194	0	12	0	0.33	217

Food	Serving	Cals	Protein (g)	Fat (g)	Carbs (g)	Fiber (g)	Sodium (mg)	Cholesterol (mg)	Calcium (mg)	Vit D (IU)	Iron (mg)	Potassium (mg)
soup, veg w/ bf broth, cnd, cond	.5 cup	66	2.42	1.56	10.7	1.3	515	1	14	0	0.79	157
soup, veg w/ bf broth, cnd, prep w/ eq volume h2o	1 cup	33	1.21	0.78	5.35	0.7	253	1	9	0	0.4	79
soup, veg, cnd, lo na, cond	.5 cup	65	2.2	0.9	12.11	2.1	385	0	20	0	0.66	433
soup, vegetarian veg, cnd, cond	.5 cup	59	1.72	1.58	9.78	0.5	516	0	17	0	0.88	171
soup, vegetarian veg, cnd, prep w/ eq volume h2o	1 cup	28	0.86	0.79	4.89	0.3	338	0	10	0	0.44	86
soup, wonton, chinese restaurant	1 cup	32	2.08	0.26	5.25	0.2	406	4	5	0	0.21	32
sour cream, fat free	1 tablespoon	74	3.1	0	15.6	0	141	9	125	0	0	129
sour cream, light	1 tablespoon	136	3.5	10.6	7.1	0	83	35	141	8	0.07	212
sour cream, reduced fat	1 tablespoon	181	7	14.1	7	0	70	35	141	10	0.06	211
sour crm, imitn, cultured	1 oz	208	2.4	19.52	6.63	0	102	0	3	0	0.39	161
sour drsng, non-butterfat, cultured, filled cream-type	1 tbsp	178	3.25	16.57	4.68	0	48	5	113	0	0.03	162
soy protein isolate	1 oz	335	88.32	3.39	0	0	1005	0	178	0	14.5	81
soy sau made from hydrolyzed veg prot	1 tbsp	60	7	0.1	7.84	0.5	6820	0	17	0	0.33	447
soy sau made from soy (tamari)	1 tbsp	60	10.51	0.1	5.57	0.8	5586	0	20	0	2.38	212
soy sau made from soy&wheat (shoyu)	1 tbsp	53	8.14	0.57	4.93	0.8	5493	0	33	0	1.45	435
soy sau made from soy&wheat (shoyu), lo na	1 tbsp	57	9.05	0.3	5.59	0.7	3598	0	30	0	1.35	352
soy sau, red na, made from hydrolyzed veg prot	1 tbsp	90	8.19	0.31	14.44	0.3	2890	0	11	0	0.43	3098
soybean, curd cheese	1 cup	151	12.5	8.1	6.9	0	20	0	188	0	5.6	199
soybeans, green, raw	1 cup	147	12.95	6.8	11.05	4.2	15	0	197	0	3.55	620
soybeans, grn, ckd, bld, drnd, w/salt	1 cup	141	12.35	6.4	11.05	4.2	250	0	145	0	2.5	539
soybeans, grn, ckd, bld, drnd, wo/salt	1 cup	141	12.35	6.4	11.05	4.2	14	0	145	0	2.5	539
soymilk (all flavors), enhanced	1 cup	45	2.94	1.99	3.45	0.4	50	0	140	47	0.49	141
soymilk (all flavors), lowfat, w/ added ca, vitamins a & d	1 cup	43	1.65	0.62	7.2	0.8	37	0	82	41	0.44	64
soymilk (all flavors), nonfat, w/ added ca, vitamins a & d	1 cup	28	2.47	0.04	4.14	0.2	57	0	116	41	0.35	105
soymilk (all flavors), unswtnd, w/ added ca, vitamins a & d	1 cup	33	2.86	1.61	1.74	0.5	37	0	124	49	0.46	120
spaghetti w/ meat sau, frz entree	1 serving	90	5.05	1.01	15.24	1.8	238	6	18	0	1.25	144
spaghetti, protein-fortified, ckd, enr (n x 6.25)	1 cup	164	8.86	0.21	30.88	2	5	0	10	0	0.72	42
spaghetti, protein-fortified, dry, enr (n x 6.25)	2 oz	374	21.78	2.23	65.65	2.4	8	0	39	0	4.15	201
spaghetti, spinach, cooked	1 cup	130	4.58	0.63	26.15		14	0	30	0	1.04	58
spaghetti, spinach, dry	2 oz	372	13.35	1.57	74.81	10.6	36	0	58	0	2.13	376
spaghetti, w/ meatballs in tomato sau, cnd	1 cup	100	4.37	4.11	11.45	2.7	280	7	29	8	1.03	217
spaghettios, spaghettios w/ meatballs	1 cup	95	4.37	2.78	12.7	1.6	238	8	60	16	1.43	282
spaghettios, spaghettios w/ sliced franks	1 cup	87	3.57	2.38	12.7	1.6	238	8	60	16	1.07	333
spanish rice mix, dry mix, prep (with canola/vegetable oil ble	1 cup	125	3.27	2.38	22.74	1.5	349		18		1.02	185
spanish rice mix, dry mix, unprep	.5 cup	363	10.62	1.62	76.45	3.1	1085		29		3.32	445
spearmint, dried	1 tsp	285	19.93	6.03	52.04	29.8	344	0	1488	0	87.47	1924
spearmint, fresh	2 leaves	44	3.29	0.73	8.41	6.8	30	0	199	0	11.87	458
spelt, ckd	1 cup	127	5.5	0.85	26.44	3.9	5	0	10	0	1.67	143
spices, basil, dried	1 tsp, leaves	233	22.98	4.07	47.75	37.7	76	0	2240	0	89.8	2630
spices, bay leaf	1 tsp, crumbled	313	7.61	8.36	74.97	26.3	23	0	834	0	43	529
spices, cardamom	1 tsp, ground	311	10.76	6.7	68.47	28	18	0	383	0	13.97	1119
spices, mustard sd, ground	1 tsp	508	26.08	36.24	28.09	12.2	13	0	266	0	9.21	738
spices, oregano, dried	1 tsp, leaves	265	9	4.28	68.92	42.5	25	0	1597	0	36.8	1260
spices, tarragon, dried	1 tsp, leaves	295	22.77	7.24	50.22	7.4	62	0	1139	0	32.3	3020
spices, thyme, dried	1 tsp, leaves	276	9.11	7.43	63.94	37	55	0	1890	0	123.6	814
spinach souffle	1 cup	172	7.89	12.95	5.9	0.7	566	118	165	31	1.19	231
spinach, ckd, bld, drnd, wo/ salt	1 cup	23	2.97	0.6	3.75	2.4	70	0	136	0	3.57	466
spinach, cnd, no salt, sol&liquids	1 cup	19	2.11	0.37	2.92	2.2	75	0	83	0	1.58	230
spinach, cnd, reg pk, drnd sol	1 cup	23	2.81	0.5	3.4	2.4	322	0	127	0	2.3	346
spinach, cnd, reg pk, sol&liquids	1 cup	19	2.11	0.37	2.92	1.6	319	0	83	0	1.58	230

Food	Serving	Cals	Protein (g)	Fat (g)	Carbs (g)	Fiber (g)	Sodium (mg)	Cholesterol (mg)	Calcium (mg)	Vit D (IU)	Iron (mg)	Potassium (mg)
spinach, frz, chopd or leaf, ckd, bld, drnd, wo/salt	.5 cup	34	4.01	0.87	4.8	3.7	97	0	153	0	1.96	302
spinach, frz, chopd or leaf, unprep	1 cup	29	3.63	0.57	4.21	2.9	74	0	129	0	1.89	346
spinach, raw	1 cup	23	2.86	0.39	3.63	2.2	79	0	99	0	2.71	558
spiny lobster, mxd sp, ckd, moist heat	3 oz	143	26.41	1.94	3.12	0	227	90	63		1.41	208
split pea soup, cnd, red na, prep w/ h2o or ready-to serve	1 cup	71	3.85	0.92	11.83	1.9	166	2	17	0	0.77	183
split pea w/ ham soup, cnd, red na, prep w/ h2o or rts	1 cup	68	4	0.7	11.4	1.9	196	3	16	0	0.7	204
squash, smmr, all var, ckd, bld, drnd, wo/salt	1 cup, sliced	20	0.91	0.31	4.31	1.4	1	0	27	0	0.36	192
squash, smmr, all var, raw	1 cup, sliced	16	1.21	0.18	3.35	1.1	2	0	15	0	0.35	262
squid, mxd sp, ckd, fried	3 oz	175	17.94	7.48	7.79	0	306	260	39		1.01	279
steelhead trout, bld, cnd (alaska native)	3 oz	159	21.11	8.26	0	0	118	59	30	604	0.64	365
steelhead trout, dried, flesh (shoshone bannock)	3 oz	382	77.27	8.06	0	0	2850	227	85	628	2.96	1720
strawberries, cnd, hvy syrup pk, sol&liquids	1 cup	92	0.56	0.26	23.53	1.7	4	0	13	0	0.49	86
strawberries, frz, swtnd, sliced	1 cup, thawed	96	0.53	0.13	25.92	1.9	3	0	11	0	0.59	98
strawberries, frz, swtnd, whl	1 cup, thawed	78	0.52	0.14	21	1.9	1	0	11	0	0.47	98
strawberries, frz, unswtnd	1 cup, thawed	35	0.43	0.11	9.13	2.1	2	0	16	0	0.75	148
strawberries, raw	1 cup, halves	32	0.67	0.3	7.68	2	1	0	16	0	0.41	153
strawberry banana smth made w/ ice & low-fat yogurt	12 fl oz	65	0.86	0.14	15.05	0.9	14	1	20	0	0.14	131
strawberry-flavor bev mix, pdr	2-3 heaping tsp	389	0.1	0.2	99.1	0	38	0	4	0	0.44	6
strawberry-flavor bev mix, pdr, prep w/ whl milk	1 cup	88	3	3.1	12.3	0	48	12	110		0.08	139
strudel, apple	1 oz	274	3.3	11.2	41.1	2.2	135	6	15	0	0.42	149
sturgeon, mxd sp, ckd, dry heat	3 oz	135	20.7	5.18	0	0	69	77	17	515	0.9	364
sturgeon, mxd sp, smoked	1 oz	173	31.2	4.4	0	0	739	80	17	642	0.93	379
submarine sndwch, bacon, lettuce, & tomato wht brd	6 inch, sub	205	10.06	6.41	26.66	1.6	354	13	210	1	2.14	186
submarine sndwch, cold cut brd w/ lettuce & tomato	6 inch, sub	213	10.52	10.04	20.43	1.2	575	27	171	7	1.81	282
submarine sndwch, ham on wht brd w/ lttc & tmt	6 inch, sub	151	9.12	2.53	22.91	1.3	396	12	169	9	1.78	367
submarine sndwch, meatball marinara on white bread	6 inch, sub	219	9.77	8.45	26.01	2.1	437	15	176	1	2.32	275
submarine sndwch, oven rstd chck wht brd lttc tmt	6 inch, sub	157	10.84	3.15	21.35	1.2	268	23	154	1	1.72	198
submarine sndwch, rst bf bread w/ lettuce & tomato	6 inch, sub	156	12.17	2.73	20.34	0.7	329	18	164	1	2.09	188
submarine sndwch, stk chs wht brd w/ chs, lttc tmt	6 inch, sub	183	12.29	5.34	21.49	1.2	444	24	183	6	2.02	183
submarine sndwch, trky brst wht brd lttc & tmt	6 inch, sub	147	9.12	2.31	22.42	1.3	317	10	169	1	1.84	253
submarine sndwch, trky rst bf hm brd w/ lttc & tmt	12 inch, sub	146	10.66	2.42	20.36	1.4	348	16	153	4	1.93	265
submarine sndwch, tuna bread w/ lettuce & tomato	6 inch, sub	218	12.33	12.04	15.95	0.7	329	28	136	21	1.57	177
succotash, (corn&limas), ckd, bld, drnd, wo/salt	1 cup	115	5.07	0.8	24.38	4.5	17	0	17	0	1.52	410
succotash, (corn&limas), cnd, w/crm style corn	1 cup	77	2.64	0.54	17.61	3	245	0	11	0	0.55	183
succotash, (corn&limas), cnd, w/whl kernel corn, sol&liquids	1 cup	63	2.6	0.49	13.98	2.6	221	0	11	0	0.53	163
succotash, (corn&limas), frz, ckd, bld, drnd, w/salt	1 cup	93	4.31	0.89	19.95	4.1	281	0	15	0	0.89	265
succotash, (corn&limas), raw	1 cup	99	5.03	1.02	19.59	3.8	4	0	18	0	1.83	369
sugar-coated almonds	1 piece	474	10	17.93	68.26	2.5	13	0	100	0	1.9	255
sugar, turbinado	1 tsp	399	0	0	99.8	0	3		12		0.37	29
sugars, brown	1 tsp, unpacked	380	0.12	0	98.09	0	28	0	83	0	0.71	133
sugars, granulated	1 packet	387	0	0	99.98	0	1	0	1	0	0.05	2

Food	Serving	Cals	Protein (g)	Fat (g)	Carbs (g)	Fiber (g)	Sodium (mg)	Cholesterol (mg)	Calcium (mg)	Vit D (IU)	Iron (mg)	Potassium (mg)
sugars, maple	1 tsp	354	0.1	0.2	90.9	0	11	0	90	0	1.61	274
sugars, powdered	1 cup, unsifted	389	0	0	99.77	0	2	0	1	0	0.06	2
sundae, caramel	1 sundae	196	4.71	5.98	31.81	0	126	16	122		0.14	205
sundae, hot fudge	1 sundae	180	3.57	5.46	30.17	0	115	13	131		0.37	250
sundae, strawberry	1 sundae	175	4.09	5.13	29.18	0	60	14	105		0.21	177
sunflower sd butter, w/salt	1 tbsp	617	17.28	55.2	23.32	5.7	331	0	64	0	4.12	576
sunflower sd butter, wo/salt	1 tbsp	617	17.28	55.2	23.32	5.7	3	0	64	0	4.12	576
sunflower sd flr, part defatted	1 cup	326	48.06	1.61	35.83	5.2	3	0	114	0	6.62	67
sunflower sd krnls from shell, dry rstd, w/ salt added	1 cup	546	19.33	49.8	15.31	9	6008	0	70	0	3.8	850
sunflower sd krnls, dried	1 cup	584	20.78	51.46	20	8.6	9	0	78	0	5.25	645
sunflower sd krnls, dry rstd, w/salt	1 cup	582	19.33	49.8	24.07	9	655	0	70	0	3.8	850
sunflower sd krnls, dry rstd, wo/salt	1 cup	582	19.33	49.8	24.07	11.1	3	0	70	0	3.8	850
sunflower sd krnls, oil rstd, w/salt	1 cup	592	20.06	51.3	22.89	10.6	733	0	87	0	4.28	483
sunflower sd krnls, oil rstd, wo/salt	1 cup	592	20.06	51.3	22.89	10.6	3	0	87	0	4.28	483
sunflower sd krnls, tstd, w/salt	1 cup	619	17.21	56.8	20.59	11.5	613	0	57	0	6.81	491
sunflower sd krnls, tstd, wo/salt	1 cup	619	17.21	56.8	20.59	11.5	3	0	57	0	6.81	491
swamp cabbage (skunk cabbage), ckd, bld, drnd, w/ salt	1 cup, chopped	20	2.08	0.24	3.7	1.9	358	0	54	0	1.32	284
swamp cabbage (skunk cabbage), ckd, bld, drnd, wo/ salt	1 cup, chopped	20	2.08	0.24	3.7	1.9	122	0	54	0	1.32	284
swamp cabbage, (skunk cabbage), raw	1 cup, chopped	19	2.6	0.2	3.14	2.1	113	0	77	0	1.67	312
sweet choc coatd fondant	1 patty, large	366	2.2	9.3	80.4	2.1	26	0	17	0	1.56	168
sweet chocolate	1 oz	507	3.9	34.2	60.4	5.5	16	0	24	0	2.76	290
sweet potato, ckd, bkd in skn, flesh, w/ salt	1 medium potato	92	2.01	0.15	20.71	3.3	246	0	38	0	0.69	475
sweet potato, ckd, bkd in skn, flesh, wo/ salt	1 cup	90	2.01	0.15	20.71	3.3	36	0	38	0	0.69	475
sweet potato, ckd, bld, wo/ skn	1 cup, mashed	76	1.37	0.14	17.72	2.5	27	0	27	0	0.72	230
sweet potato, ckd, bld, wo/ skn, w/ salt	1 cup, mashed	76	1.37	0.14	17.72	2.5	263	0	27	0	0.72	230
sweet potato, ckd, candied, home-prepared	1 piece	164	0.89	3.54	32.12	2.1	119	9	26	2	0.79	178
sweet potato, cnd, mshd	1 cup	101	1.98	0.2	23.19	1.7	75	0	30	0	1.33	210
sweet potato, cnd, syrup pk, drnd sol	1 cup	108	1.28	0.32	25.36	3	39	0	17	0	0.95	193
sweet potato, cnd, syrup pk, sol & liquids	1 cup	89	0.98	0.2	20.93	2.5	29	0	15	0	0.8	185
sweet potato, frz, ckd, bkd, w/ salt	1 cup, cubes	100	1.71	0.12	23.4	1.8	244	0	35	0	0.54	377
sweet potato, frz, ckd, bkd, wo/ salt	1 cup, cubes	100	1.71	0.12	23.4	1.8	8	0	35	0	0.54	377
sweet potato, frz, unprep	1 cup, cubes	96	1.71	0.18	22.22	1.7	6	0	37	0	0.53	365
sweet potato, raw, unprep	1 cup, cubes	86	1.57	0.05	20.12	3	55	0	30	0	0.61	337
sweet potatoes, french fr, crosscut, frz, unprep	3 oz	209	1.7	11.1	25.52	3.4	214	0	39		0.44	244
sweet potatoes, french fr, frz as packaged, salt added	12 fries	182	2.16	8.92	35.58	5.7	146	0	52	0	0.77	409
sweet rolls, cheese	1 oz	360	7.1	18.3	43.7	1.2	357	76	118		0.76	137
sweet rolls, cinn, commly prep w/ raisins	1 oz	372	6.2	16.4	50.9	2.4	304	66	72	0	1.6	111
sweet rolls, cinn, refr dough w/frstng	1 oz	333	5	12.2	51.6		765	0	31		2.44	58
sweet rolls, cinn, refr dough w/ frstng, bkd	1 oz	362	5.4	13.2	56.1		832	0	34		2.65	63
sweetener, herbal extract pdr from stevia leaf	1 packet	0	0	0	100	0	0	0	0	0	0	0
sweetener, syrup, agave	1 tsp	310	0.09	0.45	76.37	0.2	4	0	1	0	0.09	4
sweeteners, for baking, brown, contains sugar & sucralose	1 tbsp	388	0	0	97.11		11		63		1.64	130
sweeteners, for baking, contains sugar & sucralose	1 tbsp	398	0	0	99.53		2		1		0.06	2
sweeteners, sugar sub, granulated, brown	1 tsp	347	2.06	0	84.77	0.6	572		879		0.16	39
sweeteners, tabletop, asprt, eq, packets	1 tsp	365	2.17	0	89.08	0	0	0	0	0	0.04	4

Food	Serving	Cals	Protein (g)	Fat (g)	Carbs (g)	Fiber (g)	Sodium (mg)	Cholesterol (mg)	Calcium (mg)	Vit D (IU)	Iron (mg)	Potassium (mg)
sweeteners, tabletop, fructose, dry, pdr	1 cup	368	0	0	100	0	12	0	0	0	0.1	0
sweeteners, tabletop, fructose, liq	1 packet	279	0	0	76.1	0.1	2	0	1	0	0.11	0
sweeteners, tabletop, saccharin (sodium saccharin)	1 packet	360	0.94	0	89.11	0	428	0	0	0	0.04	4
sweeteners, tabletop, sucralose, splenda packets	1 packet	336	0	0	91.17	0	0	0	0	0	0	4
swisswurst pork & bf w/ swiss chs smoked	2.7 oz	307	12.69	27.37	1.6	0	827	61	74		0.72	206
swordcooked, dry heat	3 oz	172	23.45	7.93	0	0	97	78	6	666	0.45	499
syrup, cane	1 oz	269	0	0	73.14	0	58	0	13	0	3.6	63
syrup, fruit flav	1 cup	261	0	0.02	65.1	0	0	0	0	0	0.03	1
syrups, choc, fudge-type	1 cup	350	4.6	8.9	62.9	2.8	346	1	49	0	1.3	284
syrups, corn, dk	1 cup	286	0	0	77.59	0	155	0	18	0	0.37	44
syrups, corn, high-fructose	1 cup	281	0	0	76	0	2	0	0	0	0.03	0
syrups, corn, lt	1 cup	283	0	0.2	76.79	0	62	0	13	0	0	1
syrups, grenadine	1 tbsp	268	0	0	66.91	0	27	0	6	0	0.05	28
syrups, malt	1 cup	318	6.2	0	71.3	0	35	0	61		0.96	320
syrups, maple	1 tbsp	260	0.04	0.06	67.04	0	12	0	102	0	0.11	212
syrups, sorghum	1 cup	290	0	0	74.9	0	8	0	150	0	3.8	1000
syrups, sugar free	1 cup	52	0.8	0	12.13	0.7	210	0	0	0	0	0
syrups, table blends, pancake, w/ butter	1/4 cup	291	0	0.09	72.43	0	287	0	2	0	0.09	3
taco salad	1.5 cup	141	6.68	7.46	11.91		385	22	97		1.15	210
taco w/ bf, chs & lettuce, hard shell	1 taco	226	8.86	12.7	19.85	3.9	397	28	89	4	1.19	209
taco w/ bf, chs & lettuce, soft	1 taco	206	9.25	9.75	20.23	2.9	560	25	123	3	1.67	161
taco w/ chick, lettuce & chs, soft	1 taco	189	13.3	6.35	19.69	1.2	613	29	122	3	1.59	217
taffy, prepared-from-recipe	1 tamale	397	0.03	3.33	91.56	0	52	9	8		0.01	3
tamales (navajo)	1 tamale	153	6.28	6.12	18.12	3.1	427	17	29		1.22	131
tamales, masa & pork filling (hopi)	4 oz	168	13.19	4.7	18.28	3.3	298	27	18		0.66	250
tamarinds, raw	1 cup, pulp	239	2.8	0.6	62.5	5.1	28	0	74	0	2.8	628
tangerines, (mandarin oranges), raw	1 cup, sections	53	0.81	0.31	13.34	1.8	2	0	37	0	0.15	166
tapioca, pearl, dry	1 cup	358	0.19	0.02	88.69	0.9	1	0	20	0	1.58	11
taquitos, frz, bf & chs, oven-heated	1 taquito	287	9.4	12.79	33.46	2.8	456	11	97	1	2.67	174
taquitos, frz, chick & chs, oven-heated	1 taquito	284	9.21	12.54	33.63	2.9	453	13	104	3	2.47	155
tea, black, brewed, prep w/ distilled h2o	1 fl oz	1	0	0	0.3	0	0	0	0		0.01	21
tea, black, brewed, prep w/ tap h2o	1 fl oz	1	0	0	0.3	0	3	0	0	0	0.02	37
tea, black, brewed, prep w/ tap h2o, decaffeinated	1 fl oz	1	0	0	0.3	0	3	0	0	0	0.02	37
tea, black, ready to drk	16 fl oz	0	0	0	0	0	2	0	0	0	0	0
tea, black, ready to drk, decaffeinated	1 cup	38	0	0	8.75	0	8	0	11	0	0	27
tea, black, ready to drk, decaffeinated, diet	1 cup	0	0	0	0.83	0	4	0	11	0	0	27
tea, black, rtd, lemon, diet	1 cup	1	0	0	0.22	0	17	0	0	0	0	14
tea, black, rtd, lemon, swtnd	1 cup	45	0	0.22	10.8	0	3	0	4	0	0	14
tea, black, rtd, peach, diet	1 cup	1	0	0	0.25	0	5	0	1	0	0	12
tea, grn, brewed, decaffeinated	240 ml	0	0	0	0	0	0	0	0	0	0	15
tea, grn, brewed, reg	1 cup	1	0.22	0	0	0	1	0	0	0	0.02	8
tea, grn, inst, decaffei, lemon, unswtnd, fort w/ vit c	2 tbsp	378	0	0	94.45	0	0	0	2	0	0.21	169
tea, grn, ready to drk, ginseng & honey, swtnd	1 cup	30	0	0.18	7.16	0	2	0	3	0	0.02	5
tea, grn, ready to drk, unswtnd	16 fl oz	0	0	0	0	0	7	0	1	0	0	19
tea, grn, rtd, citrus, diet, fort w/ vit c	1 cup	1	0	0	0.31	0	26	0	1	0	0	13
tea, grn, rtd, diet	1 cup	0	0	0	0	0	6	0	1	0	0	5
tea, grn, rtd, swtnd	1 cup	27	0	0.22	6.2	0	21	0	1	0	0	12
tea, herb, brewed, chamomile	1 fl oz	1	0	0	0.2	0	1	0	2	0	0.08	9
tea, herb, other than chamomile, brewed	1 fl oz	1	0	0	0.2	0	1	0	2	0	0.08	9
tea, hibiscus, brewed	8 fl oz	0	0	0	0	0	4	0	8	0	0.08	20
tea, inst, decaffeinated, lemon, diet	2 tsp	338	3.3	0.6	85.4	0	412	0	21	0	8.87	2568
tea, inst, decaffeinated, lemon, swtnd	3 heaping tsp	401	0.12	0.73	98.55	0	5	0	2		0.21	169
tea, inst, decaffeinated, unswtnd	2 tsp	315	20.21	0	58.66	8.5	72	0	118	0	2.26	6040

Food	Serving	Cals	Protein (g)	Fat (g)	Carbs (g)	Fiber (g)	Sodium (mg)	Cholesterol (mg)	Calcium (mg)	Vit D (IU)	Iron (mg)	Potassium (mg)
tea, inst, lemon, diet	1 fl oz	2	0.02	0	0.44	0	6	0	3	0	0.05	14
tea, inst, lemon, swtnd, pdr	3 heaping tsp	401	0.12	0.73	98.55	0.7	5	0	2	0	0.21	169
tea, inst, lemon, swtnd, prep w/ h2o	1 cup	35	0.01	0.06	8.61	0.1	2	0	2		0.02	15
tea, inst, lemon, unswtnd	1 tsp, rounded	345	7.4	0.18	78.52	5	55	0	28	0	0.75	3453
tea, inst, lemon, w/ added vit c	3 heaping tsp	385	0.6	0.3	97.6	0	5	0	3		0.16	217
tea, inst, swtnd w/ na saccharin, lemon-flavored, pdr	2 tsp	338	3.3	0.6	85.4	0	412	0	21		8.87	2568
tea, inst, unswtnd, pdr	1 serving, 1 tsp	315	20.21	0	58.66	8.5	72	0	118	0	2.26	6040
tea, inst, unswtnd, prep w/ h2o	1 fl oz	1	0.06	0	0.17	0	4	0	3	0	0.01	18
tea, oolong, brewed	1 cup	1	0	0	0.15	0	3	0	1	0	0	12
tea, rtd, lemon, diet	1 cup	2	0	0	0.41	0	1	0	0	0	0	37
teff, unckd	1 cup	367	13.3	2.38	73.13	8	12		180		7.63	427
tempeh	1 cup	192	20.29	10.8	7.64		9	0	111	0	2.7	412
tempeh, ckd	1 cup	195	19.91	11.38	7.62		14		96	0	2.13	401
thyme, frsh	1 tsp	101	5.56	1.68	24.45	14	9	0	405	0	17.45	609
tilapia, ckd, dry heat	1 fillet	128	26.15	2.65	0	0	56	57	14	150	0.69	380
toaster pastries, brown-sugar-cinnamon	1 oz	370	4.06	7.98	72.64	2.3	361		293		5.62	105
toaster pastries, fruit	1 oz	388	4.2	9.95	70.32	1	334	0	16	0	5.51	102
toaster pastries, fruit, frstd	1 pastry	385	4.01	9.02	71.83	1.8	311	0	12	0	4.35	86
toaster pstrs, frt, tstd (incl appl, blueberry, cherry, strawberry)	1 pastry	409	4.7	11.03	72.7	1	354		11		3.92	81
toffee, prepared-from-recipe	1 piece	560	1.07	32.75	64.72	0	135	104	34		0.03	51
tofu, ex firm, prep w/nigari	.2 block	83	9.98	5.26	1.18	1	4	0	282	0	2.04	130
tofu, firm, prep w/ca sulfate&magnesium chloride (nigari)	.5 cup	78	9.04	4.17	2.85	0.9	12	0	201	0	1.61	148
tofu, fried	1 oz	270	18.82	20.18	8.86	3.9	16	0	372	0	4.87	146
tofu, fried, prep w/ca sulfate	1 block	270	18.82	20.18	8.86	3.9	16	0	961	0	4.87	146
tofu, hard, prep w/nigari	.25 block	145	12.68	9.99	4.39	0.6	2	0	345	0	2.75	146
tofu, raw, firm, prep w/ca sulfate	.5 cup	144	17.27	8.72	2.78	2.3	14	0	683	0	2.66	237
tofu, raw, reg, prep w/ca sulfate	.5 cup	76	8.08	4.78	1.87	0.3	7	0	350	0	5.36	121
tofu, salted&fermented (fuyu)	1 block	116	8.92	8	4.38		2873	0	46	0	1.98	75
tofu, salted&fermented (fuyu), prep w/ca sulfate	1 block	116	8.15	8	5.15		2873	0	1229	0	1.98	75
tofu, soft, prep w/ca sulfate&magnesium chloride (nigari)	1 block	61	7.17	3.69	1.18	0.2	8	0	111	0	1.11	120
tomatillos, raw	1 block	32	0.96	1.02	5.84	1.9	1	0	7	0	0.62	268
tomato juc, cnd, w/salt	1 cup	17	0.85	0.29	3.53	0.4	253	0	10	0	0.39	217
tomato juc, cnd, wo/ salt added	1 cup	17	0.85	0.29	3.53	0.4	10	0	10	0	0.39	217
tomato powder	100 g	302	12.91	0.44	74.68	16.5	134	0	166	0	4.56	1927
tomato products, cnd, paste, wo/ salt added	.25 cup	82	4.32	0.47	18.91	4.1	59	0	36	0	2.98	1014
tomato products, cnd, puree, w/salt	1 cup	38	1.65	0.21	8.98	1.9	202	0	18	0	1.78	439
tomato products, cnd, puree, wo/salt	1 cup	38	1.65	0.21	8.98	1.9	28	0	18	0	1.78	439
tomato products, cnd, sau	1 cup	24	1.2	0.3	5.31	1.5	474	0	14	0	0.96	297
tomato products, cnd, sau, spanish style	1 cup	33	1.44	0.27	7.24	1.4	472	0	17	0	3.48	369
tomato products, cnd, sau, w/ herbs&chs	.5 cup	59	2.13	1.93	10.24	2.2	543	3	37	0	0.87	356
tomato products, cnd, sau, w/ mushrooms	1 cup	35	1.45	0.13	8.43	1.5	452	0	13		0.89	380
tomato products, cnd, sau, w/onions	1 cup	42	1.56	0.19	9.94	1.8	551	0	17	0	0.93	413
tomato products, cnd, sau, w/onions, grn peppers, &celery	1 cup	41	0.94	0.74	8.77	1.4	368	0	13	0	0.76	398
tomato products, cnd, sau, w/tomato tidbits	1 cup	32	1.32	0.39	7.09	1.4	15	0	10	0	0.68	373
tomato sau, cnd, no salt added	1 cup	24	1.2	0.3	5.31	1.5	11	0	14	0	0.96	297
tomato&veg juc, lo na	1 cup	22	0.6	0.1	4.59	0.8	58	0	11	0	0.42	193
tomatoes, crushed, canned	.5 cup	32	1.64	0.28	7.29	1.9	186	0	34	0	1.3	293
tomatoes, green, raw	1 cup	23	1.2	0.2	5.1	1.1	13	0	13	0	0.51	204
tomatoes, orange, raw	1 cup, chopped	16	1.16	0.19	3.18	0.9	42	0	5	0	0.47	212

237

Food	Serving	Cals	Protein (g)	Fat (g)	Carbs (g)	Fiber (g)	Sodium (mg)	Cholesterol (mg)	Calcium (mg)	Vit D (IU)	Iron (mg)	Potassium (mg)
tomatoes, red, ripe, ckd	1 cup	18	0.95	0.11	4.01	0.7	11	0	11	0	0.68	218
tomatoes, red, ripe, ckd, stwd	1 cup	79	1.96	2.68	13.05	1.7	455	0	26	0	1.06	247
tomatoes, red, ripe, ckd, w/ salt	1 cup	18	0.95	0.11	4.01	0.7	247	0	11	0	0.68	218
tomatoes, red, ripe, cnd, packed in tomato juc	1 cup	16	0.79	0.25	3.47	1.9	115	0	33	0	0.57	191
tomatoes, red, ripe, cnd, packed in tomato juc, no salt added	1 cup	16	0.79	0.25	3.47	1.9	10	0	33	0	0.57	191
tomatoes, red, ripe, cnd, stwd	1 cup	26	0.91	0.19	6.19	1	221	0	34	0	1.33	207
tomatoes, red, ripe, cnd, w/grn chilies	1 cup	15	0.69	0.08	3.62		401	0	20	0	0.26	107
tomatoes, red, ripe, raw, year rnd average	1 cup	18	0.88	0.2	3.89	1.2	5	0	10	0	0.27	237
tomatoes, sun-dried	1 cup	258	14.11	2.97	55.76	12.3	107	0	110	0	9.09	3427
tomatoes, sun-dried, packed in oil, drnd	1 cup	213	5.06	14.08	23.33	5.8	266	0	47	0	2.68	1565
tomatoes, yellow, raw	1 cup, chopped	15	0.98	0.26	2.98	0.7	23	0	11	0	0.49	258
tonic water	1 fl oz	34	0	0	8.8	0	12	0	1	0	0.01	0
toppings, butterscotch or caramel	2 tbsp	216	1.21	0	57.01	0	341	0	49	0	0	66
toppings, marshmllw crm	1 oz	322	0.8	0.3	79	0.1	80	0	3	0	0.22	5
toppings, nuts in syrup	1 cup	448	4.5	22	58.08	2.3	42	0	35	0	1.05	151
toppings, pineapple	1 cup	253	0.1	0.1	66.4	0.4	42	0	6	0	0.12	43
toppings, strawberry	2 tbsp	254	0.2	0.1	66.3	0.7	21	0	6	0	0.28	51
tortellini, pasta w/ chs filling, fresh-refrigerated	.75 cup	307	13.5	7.23	47	1.9	406	42	152	0	1.5	89
tortilla chips, nacho cheese	1 oz	519	7.36	27.42	60.81	5.1	691	0	137	0	1.16	223
tortilla chips, plain	1 oz	472	7.1	20.68	67.78	5.4	328	0	106	0	1.52	182
tortilla chips, yellow, plain, salted	1 oz	497	6.62	22.33	67.38	4.7	310	0	104	0	1.32	206
tortilla, incl pln & from mutton sndwch (navajo)	1 serving	237	7.28	0.95	49.94	2.4	482		70		3.81	105
tortillas, rtb or -fry, corn	1 oz	218	5.7	2.85	44.64	6.3	45	0	81	0	1.23	186
tortillas, rtb or -fry, corn, wo/ salt	1 oz	222	5.7	2.5	46.6	5.2	11	0	175		1.4	154
tortillas, rtb or -fry, flr, refr	1 tortilla	306	8.2	7.99	49.43	3.5	736	0	146	0	3.63	125
tortillas, rtb or -fry, flr, shelf stable	1 tortilla	297	8.01	7.58	49.27	2.4	742	0	163	0	3.32	133
tortillas, rtb or -fry, flr, wo/ ca	1 oz	325	8.7	7.1	55.6	3.3	478	0	39		3.3	131
tortillas, rtb or -fry, whl wheat	1 tortilla	310	9.76	9.76	45.89	9.8	512	0	244	0	2.63	262
tostada shells, corn	1 piece	474	6.15	23.38	64.43	5.8	657		76		1.53	237
trail mix, reg, unsalted	1 cup	462	13.8	29.4	44.9		10	0	78		3.05	685
trail mix, reg, w/choc chips, salted nuts&seeds	1 cup	484	14.2	31.9	44.9	5	121	4	109	0	3.39	648
trail mix, reg, w/choc chips, unsalted nuts&seeds	1 cup	484	14.2	31.9	44.9		27	0	109		3.39	648
trail mix, regular	1 cup	462	13.8	29.4	44.9		229	0	78		3.05	685
trail mix, tropical	1 cup	442	6.3	17.1	65.6		95	0	57		2.64	709
tropical punch, rtd	1 cup	10	0	0	2.5	0	13	0	0	0	0	0
trout, brook, raw, new york state	1 filet	110	21.23	2.73	0		45	60	25		0.38	417
trout, mxd sp, ckd, dry heat	1 fillet	190	26.63	8.47	0	0	67	74	55		1.92	463
trout, rainbow, farmed, ckd, dry heat	1 fillet	168	23.8	7.38	0	0	61	70	30	759	0.36	450
trout, rainbow, wild, ckd, dry heat	1 fillet	150	22.92	5.82	0	0	56	69	86		0.38	448
truffles, prepared-from-recipe	1 piece	510	6.21	33.76	44.88	2.5	68	53	157		1.75	297
tuna salad	3 oz	187	16.04	9.26	9.41	0	402	13	17		1	178
tuna, fresh, bluefin, raw	3 oz	144	23.33	4.9	0	0	39	38	8	227	1.02	252
tuna, fresh, skipjack, raw	3 oz	103	22	1.01	0	0	37	47	29		1.25	407
tuna, fresh, yellowfin, raw	1 oz, boneless	109	24.4	0.49	0	0	45	39	4	69	0.77	441
tuna, frsh, bluefin, ckd, dry heat	3 oz	184	29.91	6.28	0	0	50	49	10		1.31	323
tuna, lt, cnd in h2o, drnd sol	1 oz	86	19.44	0.96	0	0	247	36	17	47	1.63	179
tuna, lt, cnd in h2o, wo/salt, drnd sol	3 oz	116	25.51	0.82	0	0	50	30	11		1.53	237
tuna, lt, cnd in oil, drnd sol	1 cup, solid or chunks	198	29.13	8.21	0	0	416	18	13	269	1.39	207
tuna, lt, cnd in oil, wo/salt, drnd sol	3 oz	198	29.13	8.21	0	0	50	18	13		1.39	207
tuna, skipjack, frsh, ckd, dry heat	3 oz	132	28.21	1.29	0	0	47	60	37		1.6	522
tuna, white, cnd in h2o, drnd sol	3 oz	128	23.62	2.97	0	0	377	42	14	80	0.97	237
tuna, white, cnd in h2o, wo/salt, drnd sol	3 oz	128	23.62	2.97	0	0	50	42	14		0.97	237

Food	Serving	Cals	Protein (g)	Fat (g)	Carbs (g)	Fiber (g)	Sodium (mg)	Cholesterol (mg)	Calcium (mg)	Vit D (IU)	Iron (mg)	Potassium (mg)
tuna, white, cnd in oil, drnd sol	3 oz	186	26.53	8.08	0	0	396	31	4		0.65	333
tuna, white, cnd in oil, wo/salt, drnd sol	3 oz	186	26.53	8.08	0	0	50	31	4		0.65	333
tuna, yellowfin, frsh, ckd, dry heat	3 oz	130	29.15	0.59	0	0	54	47	4	82	0.92	527
turkey and gravy, frozen	3 oz	67	5.88	2.63	4.61	0	554	18	14		0.93	61
turkey bacon, microwaved	1 slice	368	29.5	25.87	4.24	0	2021	153	163	50	2.63	666
turkey breast, lo salt, prepackaged or deli, luncheon meat	1 slice	109	21.81	0.83	3.51	0.5	772	44	8	2	0.63	211
turkey breast, pre-basted, meat&skn, ckd, rstd	3 oz	126	22.16	3.46	0	0	397	42	9		0.66	248
turkey breast, sliced, prepackaged	1 slice	106	14.81	3.77	2.2	0	898	49	14	6	0.42	371
turkey from whl, lt meat, meat & skn, ckd, rstd	1 serving	177	29.55	5.57	0.05	0	101	89	11	14	0.8	248
turkey from whl, lt meat, meat & skn, w/ added soln, ckd, rstd	3 oz	157	26.52	5.64	0	0	237	76	14	14	0.6	250
turkey from whl, lt meat, meat & skn, w/ added soln, raw	4 oz	147	20.02	7.42	0.14	0	195	60	14	11	0.54	220
turkey from whl, lt meat, meat only, w/ added soln, ckd, rstd	3 oz	127	26.97	2.08	0	0	238	69	13	10	0.55	249
turkey from whl, neck, meat only, ckd, simmrd	3 oz	162	22.48	7.36	0	0	246	128	58	12	1.18	114
turkey ham, sliced, ex ln, prepackaged or deli-sliced	1 cup, pieces	124	19.6	3.8	2.93	0	1038	67	5	2	1.35	299
turkey pot pie, frz entree	1 package, yields	176	6.5	8.8	17.7	1.1	350	16			1	
turkey sausage, frsh, ckd	1link	196	23.89	10.44	0	0	665	92	22		1.49	298
turkey sausage, red fat, brown&serve, ckd	1 cup	204	17	10.3	10.92	0.3	721	58	31	17	1.8	207
turkey stks, breaded, battered, fried	2.25 oz	279	14.2	16.9	17		838	64	14		2.2	260
turkey thigh, pre-basted, meat&skn, ckd, rstd	3 oz	157	18.8	8.54	0	0	437	62	8		1.51	241
turkey white rotisserie deli cut	1.69 oz	112	13.5	3	7.7	0.4	1200	55	16		2.2	349
turkey, all classes, back, meat&skn, ckd, rstd	1 cup, chopped or diced	244	26.59	14.38	0.16	0	73	91	33	1	2.19	260
turkey, all classes, breast, meat&skn, ckd, rstd	3 oz	189	28.71	7.41	0	0	63	74	21		1.4	288
turkey, all classes, leg, meat&skn, ckd, rstd	3 oz	208	27.87	9.82	0	0	77	85	32	4	2.3	280
turkey, all classes, lt meat, ckd, rstd	3 oz	147	30.13	2.08	0	0	99	80	9	10	0.71	249
turkey, all classes, wing, meat&skn, ckd, rstd	3 oz	229	27.38	12.43	0	0	61	81	24	4	1.46	266
turkey, back, from whl bird, meat & skn, w/ added soln, rstd	3 oz	205	25.8	11.36	0	0	237	87	15	21	0.68	252
turkey, back, from whl bird, meat only, rstd	3 oz	173	27.71	6.04	0	0	104	128	17	10	1.43	227
turkey, back, from whl bird, meat only, w/ added soln, rstd	3 oz	127	26.97	2.08	0	0	238	69	13	10	0.55	249
turkey, breast, from whl bird, meat only, rstd	3 oz	147	30.13	2.08	0	0	99	80	9	10	0.71	249
turkey, breast, from whl bird, meat only, w/ added soln, rstd	3 oz	127	26.97	2.08	0	0	238	69	13	10	0.55	249
turkey, breast, smoked, lemon pepper flavor, 97% fat-free	1 slice	95	20.9	0.69	1.31	0	1160	48				
turkey, cnd, meat only, w/broth	1 cup, drained	169	23.68	6.86	1.47	0	518	66	12	11	1.86	224
turkey, diced, lt&dk meat, seasoned	1 oz	138	18.7	6	1	0	850	55	1		1.8	310
turkey, dk meat from whl, meat & skn, ckd, rstd	3 oz	206	27.27	9.95	0.07	0	105	134	17	15	1.45	228
turkey, dk meat from whl, meat & skn, w/ added soln, ckd, rstd	3 oz	199	25.55	10.81	0	0	206	110	17	16	1.08	232
turkey, dk meat, meat only, w/ added soln, ckd, rstd	3 oz	158	26.1	6	0	0	201	105	16	10	1.07	227
turkey, drumstk, from whl bird, meat only, rstd	3 oz	139	30.13	2.08	0	0	99	80	9	10	0.71	249

Food	Serving	Cals	Protein (g)	Fat (g)	Carbs (g)	Fiber (g)	Sodium (mg)	Cholesterol (mg)	Calcium (mg)	Vit D (IU)	Iron (mg)	Potassium (mg)
turkey, drumstk, from whl bird, meat only, w/ added soln, rstd	3 oz	158	26.1	6	0	0	201	105	16	10	1.07	227
turkey, young hen, skn only, ckd, rstd	3 oz	482	19.03	44.45	0	0	44	106	32		1.82	155
turkey&pork sausage, frsh, bulk, patty or link, ckd	1 cup, cooked	307	22.7	23	0.7	0	878	84	32	79	1.62	337
turmeric, ground	1 tsp	312	9.68	3.25	67.14	22.7	27	0	168	0	55	2080
turnip greens, raw	1 cup, chopped	32	1.5	0.3	7.13	3.2	40	0	190	0	1.1	296
turnip grns, ckd, bld, drnd, w/salt	1 cup, chopped	20	1.14	0.23	4.36	3.5	265	0	137	0	0.8	203
turnip grns, ckd, bld, drnd, wo/salt	1 cup, chopped	20	1.14	0.23	4.36	3.5	29	0	137	0	0.8	203
turnips, frz, ckd, bld, drnd, w/salt	1 cup	21	1.53	0.24	3.73	2	272	0	32	0	0.98	182
turnips, frz, ckd, bld, drnd, wo/salt	1 cup	23	1.53	0.24	4.35	2	36	0	32	0	0.98	182
turnips, raw	1 cup, cubes	28	0.9	0.1	6.43	1.8	67	0	30	0	0.3	191
turnover, cheese-filled, tomato-based sau, frz, unprep	1 serving, 4.5 oz	235	10.24	9.45	27.29	1.6	598	20	276	5	1.85	179
turnover, chicken- or turkey-, & vegetable-filled, red fat, frz	1 turnover	168	7.87	5.51	21.74	3.1	276	16	157	3	2.13	167
turnover, filled w/ egg, meat & chs, frz	1 turnover	228	7.87	12.6	20.67	0.8	378	31	79	15	2.13	177
turnover, meat- & cheese-filled, tomato-based sau, red fat, frz	1 turnover	215	9.45	5.51	31.89	0.8	378	20	197	5	2.13	117
vanilla extract	1 tsp	288	0.06	0.06	12.65	0	9	0	11	0	0.12	148
vanilla, lt, soft-serve ice crm, w/ cone	3 oz	163	4.24	4.86	26.36	0.1	81	15	129	0	0.35	193
veal, australian, shank, hind, bone-in, ln & fat	3 oz	144	19.78	7.2	0	0	95	60	16		2.95	
veal, breast, fat, ckd	1 oz	521	9.4	53.35	0	0	49	95	6		0.45	181
veal, breast, plate half, bnless, ln&fat, ckd, brsd	3 oz	282	25.93	18.95	0		64	112	8		0.75	266
veal, breast, point half, bnless, ln&fat, ckd, brsd	3 oz	248	28.23	14.16	0		66	114	9		0.79	278
veal, breast, whl, bnless, ln, ckd, brsd	3 oz	218	30.32	9.8	0		68	116	9		0.83	289
veal, breast, whl, bnless, ln&fat, ckd, brsd	3 oz	266	26.97	16.77	0		65	113	9		0.77	272
veal, comp of rtl cuts, fat, ckd	3 oz	642	9.42	66.74	0	0	57	73	4		1	173
veal, comp of rtl cuts, ln, ckd	3 oz	196	31.9	6.58	0	0	89	118	24	0	1.16	338
veal, comp of rtl cuts, ln&fat, ckd	3 oz	231	30.1	11.39	0	0	87	114	22	0	1.15	325
veal, cubed for stew (leg&shldr), ln, ckd, brsd	3 oz	188	34.94	4.31	0	0	93	145	29		1.44	342
veal, foreshank, osso buco, ln & fat, ckd, brsd	3 oz	182	27.94	7.77	0.11	0	90	92	22	42	2	201
veal, foreshank, osso buco, ln, ckd, brsd	3 oz	157	29.12	4.51	0	0	90	92	21	33	2.06	205
veal, ground, ckd, brld	3 oz	172	24.38	7.56	0	0	83	103	17	0	0.99	337
veal, ground, ckd, pan-fried	3 oz	215	25.83	11.78	1.51	0	146	77	18	55	1.5	245
veal, ground, raw	3 oz	197	18.58	13.06	0	0	103	49	12	51	1.37	198
veal, leg (top rnd), ln, ckd, brsd	3 oz	203	36.71	5.09	0	0	67	135	9		1.32	387
veal, loin, chop, ln & fat, ckd, grilled	3 oz	198	28.04	9.48	0.16	0	86	79	17	45	0.82	229
veal, rib, ln, ckd, brsd	3 oz	218	34.44	7.81	0	0	99	144	24	0	1.45	318
veal, rib, ln, ckd, rstd	3 oz	177	25.76	7.44	0	0	97	115	12		0.96	311
veal, rib, ln&fat, ckd, brsd	3 oz	251	32.43	12.53	0	0	95	139	22	0	1.41	306
veal, rib, ln&fat, ckd, rstd	3 oz	228	23.96	13.96	0	0	92	110	11		0.97	295
veal, shank (fore&hind), ln, ckd, brsd	3 oz	177	32.22	4.33	0	0	94	126	34		1.26	309
veal, shank (fore&hind), ln&fat, ckd, brsd	3 oz	191	31.54	6.2	0		93	124	33		1.25	305
veal, shldr, arm, ln, ckd, brsd	3 oz	201	35.73	5.33	0	0	90	155	30		1.41	347
veal, sirloin, ln, ckd, brsd	3 oz	204	33.96	6.51	0	0	81	113	19		1.23	339
veal, sirloin, ln, ckd, rstd	3 oz	168	26.32	6.22	0	0	85	104	14		0.91	365
veal, sirloin, ln&fat, ckd, brsd	3 oz	252	31.26	13.14	0	0	79	108	17		1.2	321
veal, sirloin, ln&fat, ckd, rstd	3 oz	202	25.14	10.45	0	0	83	102	13	0	0.92	351
veg & fruit juc blend, w/ added vitamins a, c, e	8 oz	46	0.3	0.01	11.15	0	29	0	8	0	0.31	101
veg & fruit juc drk, red cal, w/ low-cal swtnr, add vit c	1 serving	4	0	0	1.1	0	14	0	8	0	0.3	24

Food	Serving	Cals	Protein (g)	Fat (g)	Carbs (g)	Fiber (g)	Sodium (mg)	Cholesterol (mg)	Calcium (mg)	Vit D (IU)	Iron (mg)	Potassium (mg)
veg oil sprd, 37% fat, unspec oils, w/ salt, w/ added vitamin d	1 tbsp	339	0.51	37.77	0.66	0	589	0	6	429	0.02	34
veg oil sprd, 60% fat, stick/tub/ bottle, wo/ salt	1 tbsp	533	0.17	59.81	0.86	0	2	1	21	0	0	30
veg oil sprd, 60% fat, stick/tub/bottle, wo/ salt, w/vit d	1 tbsp	542	0.17	59.81	0.86	0	2	1	21	429	0	30
veg oil sprd, 60% fat, stk, w/ salt, w/ added vitamin d	1 tbsp	537	0.12	60.39	0.69	0	785	0	21	429	0	30
veg oil sprd, 60% fat, tub, w/ salt, w/ added vitamin d	1 tbsp	533	0.17	59.81	0.86	0	785	1	21	429	0	30
veg oil sprd, unspec oils, approx 37% fat, w/ salt	1 tbsp	339	0.51	37.77	0.66	0	589	0	6	0	0.02	34
veg-oil sprd, stick/tub/bottle, 60% fat, w/ added vitamin d	1 tbsp	535	0.6	59.17	0	0	785	1	21	429	0	30
vegetable & fruit juc drk, w/ added nutr	8 fl oz	29	0.04	0.01	7.47	0	21	0	3	0	0.04	19
vegetable juc cocktail, cnd	1 cup	22	0.93	0.31	3.87	0.5	169	0	14	0	0.28	185
vegetable juc cocktail, lo na, cnd	1 cup	19	0.91	0.32	3.83	0.5	55	0	15	0	0.29	204
vegetable juc, bolthouse farms, daily grns	1 cup	31	0.49	0.04	8.13	1.2	15	0	110	0	3.85	224
vegetable oil-butter sprd, red cal	1 tbsp	465	0	53	0	0	581	54	6	0	0.04	6
vegetable oil, palm kernel	1 tablespoon	862	0	100	0	0	0	0	0	0	0	0
vegetables, mxd (corn, lima bns, peas, grn bns, crrt) cnd, no salt	1 cup	37	1.4	0.2	7.31	3.1	26	0	21	0	0.65	138
vegetables, mxd, cnd, drnd sol	1 cup	49	2.59	0.25	9.26	3	214	0	27	0	1.05	291
vegetables, mxd, cnd, sol&liquids	1 cup	36	1.42	0.25	7.13	3.8	224	0	21	0	0.65	138
vegetables, mxd, frz, ckd, bld, drnd, w/salt	.5 cup	60	2.86	0.15	13.09	4.4	271	0	25	0	0.82	169
vegetables, mxd, frz, ckd, bld, drnd, wo/salt	.5 cup	65	2.86	0.15	13.09	4.4	35	0	25	0	0.82	169
vegetables, mxd, frz, unprep	10 oz	72	3.33	0.52	13.47	4	47	0	25	0	0.95	212
vegetarian fillets	1 fillet	290	23	18	9	6.1	490	0	95	0	2	600
vegetarian meatloaf or patties	1 slice	197	21	9	8	4.6	550	0	29	0	2.1	180
veggie burgers or soyburgers unprep	1 pattie	177	15.7	6.3	14.27	4.9	569	5	136	0	2.41	333
vermicelli, made from soy	1 cup	331	0.1	0.1	82.32	3.9	4	0	55	0	1.81	3
vinegar, balsamic	1 tbsp	88	0.49	0	17.03	0	23		27		0.72	112
vinegar, cider	1 tbsp	21	0	0	0.93	0	5	0	7	0	0.2	73
vinegar, distilled	1 tbsp	18	0	0	0.04	0	2	0	6	0	0.03	2
vinegar, red wine	1 tbsp	19	0.04	0	0.27	0	8		6		0.45	39
waffle, bttrmlk, frz, rth, microwaved	1 waffle	289	6.92	9.4	44.16	2.4	663	16	125		6.53	110
waffle, bttrmlk, frz, rth, tstd	1 oz	309	7.42	9.49	48.39	2.6	710	13	299	0	6.59	138
waffle, pln, frz, rth, microwave	1 waffle	298	6.71	9.91	45.41	2.4	682	16	197		5.81	148
waffles, bttrmlk, frz, rth	1 waffle, square	273	6.58	9.22	41.05	2.2	621	15	279		6.04	126
waffles, choc chip, frz, rth	2 waffles	297	5.8	10.1	45.68	1.5	529	21	357	2	6.4	74
waffles, gluten-free, frz, rth	1 waffle	263	2.72	8.84	43.05	1.4	505	0	40	0	0.63	124
waffles, pln, frz, ready -to-heat, tstd	1 oz	312	7.19	9.61	49.29	2.4	730	15	307	0	6.91	144
waffles, pln, frz, rth	1 oz	285	6.47	9.7	42.98	2.2	638	14	308		5.61	125
waffles, pln, prep from recipe	1 oz	291	7.9	14.1	32.9		511	69	255		2.31	159
waffles, whl wheat, lowfat, frz, rth	1 serving, 2 waffles	257	7.14	3.57	49.16	4.3	557	0	143	0	6.43	164
walblack, dried	1 cup, chopped	619	24.06	59.33	9.58	6.8	2	0	61	0	3.12	523
waldry rstd, w/ salt added	1 oz	643	14.29	60.71	17.86	7.1	643	0	71	0	2.57	459
walenglish	1 cup, chopped	654	15.23	65.21	13.71	6.7	2	0	98	0	2.91	441
walglazed	1 oz	500	8.28	35.71	47.59	3.6	446	0	71		1.29	232
wasabi	1 tablespoon	292	2.23	10.9	46.13	6.1	3390	0	41	0	0.5	182
water w/ added vit & min, bottles, swtnd, ast fruit flavors	8 fl oz	22	0	0	5.49	0	0	0	17	0	0	0
water, tap, drinking	1 fl oz	0	0	0	0	0	4	0	3	0	0	0
waterchestchinese, (matai), raw	.5 cup, slices	97	1.4	0.1	23.94	3	14	0	11	0	0.06	584
waterchestchinese, cnd, sol&liquids	.5 cup, slices	50	0.88	0.06	12.3	2.5	8	0	4	0	0.87	118
watercress, raw	1 cup, chopped	11	2.3	0.1	1.29	0.5	41	0	120	0	0.2	330

Food	Serving	Cals	Protein (g)	Fat (g)	Carbs (g)	Fiber (g)	Sodium (mg)	Cholesterol (mg)	Calcium (mg)	Vit D (IU)	Iron (mg)	Potassium (mg)
watermelon sd krnls, dried	1 cup	557	28.33	47.37	15.31		99	0	54	0	7.28	648
watermelon, raw	1 cup, balls	30	0.61	0.15	7.55	0.4	1	0	7	0	0.24	112
wheat bran, crude	1 cup	216	15.55	4.25	64.51	42.8	2	0	73	0	10.57	1182
wheat flour, whole-grain	1 cup	340	13.21	2.5	71.97	10.7	2	0	34	0	3.6	363
wheat flours, bread, unenr	1 cup, unsifted, dipped	361	11.98	1.66	72.53	2.4	2	0	15	0	0.9	100
wheat flr, white, all-purpose, enr, unbleached	1 cup	364	10.33	0.98	76.31	2.7	2	0	15	0	4.64	107
wheat flr, white, all-purpose, self-rising, enr	1 cup	354	9.89	0.97	74.22	2.7	1193	0	338	0	4.67	124
wheat flr, white, all-purpose, unenr	1 cup	364	10.33	0.98	76.31	2.7	2	0	15	0	1.17	107
wheat flr, white, bread, enr	1 cup	361	11.98	1.66	72.53	2.4	2	0	15	0	4.41	100
wheat flr, white, cake, enr	1 cup, unsifted, dipped	362	8.2	0.86	78.03	1.7	2	0	14	0	7.32	105
wheat flr, white, tortilla mix, enr	1 cup	405	9.66	10.63	67.14		677	0	205	0	7.05	100
wheat flr, whole-grain, soft wheat	1 cup	332	9.61	1.95	74.48	13.1	3	0	33	0	3.71	394
wheat, puffed, fort	1 cup	364	14.7	1.2	79.6	4.4	4	0	28		31.7	348
wheat, sprouted	1 cup	198	7.49	1.27	42.53	1.1	16	0	28	0	2.14	169
whey prot pdr isolate	3 scoop	359	58.14	1.16	29.07	0	372	12	698	0	1.26	872
whipped crm sub, dietetic, made from pdr mix	1 cup	100	0.9	6	10.6	0	106	0	3	0	0.01	26
whipped topping, frz, lofat	1 cup	224	3	13.1	23.6	0	72	2	71	0	0.1	101
whiskey sour	1 fl oz	149	0	0.03	13.17	0	20	0	1		0.08	5
whiskey sour mix, bttld	1 fl oz	87	0.1	0.1	21.4	0	102	0	2	0	0.11	28
whiskey sour mix, bttld, w/ k&na	1 fl oz	84	0.1	0.1	21.4	0	33	0	2		0.11	7
whiskey sour mix, pdr	1 packet	383	0.6	0.1	97.3	0	274	0	272		0.39	19
whiskey, 86 proof	1 fl oz	250	0	0	0.1	0	0	0	0		0.02	1
white choc	3 oz	539	5.87	32.09	59.24	0.2	90	21	199	0	0.24	286
whitemxd sp, ckd, dry heat	3 oz	172	24.47	7.51	0	0	65	77	33		0.47	406
whitemxd sp, smoked	1 cup	108	23.4	0.93	0	0	1019	33	18	512	0.5	423
whiting, mxd sp, ckd, dry heat	1 fillet	116	23.48	1.69	0	0	132	84	62	73	0.42	434
wild rice, cooked	1 cup	101	3.99	0.34	21.34	1.8	3	0	3	0	0.6	101
wine, cooking	1 tsp	50	0.5	0	6.3	0	626	0	9	0	0.4	88
wine, dssrt, dry	1 fl oz	152	0.2	0	11.67	0	9	0	8		0.24	92
wine, dssrt, swt	1 fl oz	160	0.2	0	13.69	0	9	0	8	0	0.24	92
wine, non-alcoholic	1 fl oz	6	0.5	0	1.1	0	7	0	9	0	0.4	88
wine, rose	1 fl oz	83	0.36	0	3.8	0	5	0	10	0	0.2	59
wine, table, all	5 fl oz	83	0.07	0	2.72	0	5	0	8	0	0.37	99
wine, table, red	1 fl oz	85	0.07	0	2.61	0	4	0	8	0	0.46	127
wine, table, white	1 fl oz	82	0.07	0	2.6	0	5	0	9	0	0.27	71
wonton wrappers (incl egg roll wrappers)	1 oz	291	9.8	1.5	57.9	1.8	572	9	47		3.36	82
yam, ckd, bld, drnd, or bkd, w/salt	1 cup, cubes	114	1.49	0.14	26.99	3.9	244	0	14	0	0.52	670
yam, ckd, bld, drnd, or bkd, wo/salt	1 cup, cubes	116	1.49	0.14	27.48	3.9	8	0	14	0	0.52	670
yam, raw	1 cup, cubes	118	1.53	0.17	27.88	4.1	9	0	17	0	0.54	816
yel grn colored citrus soft drk w/ caffeine	16 fl oz	49	0	0	12.83	0	18	0	13	0	0.02	2
yellow rice w/ seasoning, dry packet mix, unprep	2 oz	343	7.02	1.75	74.68	1.8	1316	0	35	0	2.53	801
yellowtail, mxd sp, ckd, dry heat	.5 fillet	187	29.67	6.72	0	0	50	71	29		0.63	538
yellowtail, mxd sp, raw	3 oz	146	23.14	5.24	0	0	39	55	23		0.49	420
yogurt parfait, lowfat, w/ fruit & granola	1 parfait	84	3.36	1.01	15.86	1.1	49	3	105	4	0.49	189
yogurt, choc, nonfat milk	6 oz	112	3.53	0	23.53	1.2	135	1	88	0	0.42	339
yogurt, choc, nonfat milk, fort w/ vitamin d	6 oz	112	3.53	0	23.53	1.2	135	1	88	47	0.42	339
yogurt, fruit var, non-fat	6 oz	95	4.4	0.2	19	0	58	2	152	0	0.07	194
yogurt, fruit var, nonfat, fort w/ vitamin d	6 oz	95	4.4	0.2	19	0	58	2	152	52	0.07	194
yogurt, fruit, lofat, 10 grams prot per 8 oz	6 oz	102	4.37	1.08	19.05	0	58	4	152	1	0.07	195

Food	Serving	Cals	Protein (g)	Fat (g)	Carbs (g)	Fiber (g)	Sodium (mg)	Cholesterol (mg)	Calcium (mg)	Vit D (IU)	Iron (mg)	Potassium (mg)
yogurt, fruit, lofat, 10 grams prot per 8 oz, fort w/ vitamin d	6 oz	102	4.37	1.08	19.05	0	58	4	152	52	0.07	195
yogurt, fruit, lofat, 11 grams prot per 8 oz	6 oz	105	4.86	1.41	18.6	0	65	6	169		0.07	216
yogurt, fruit, lofat, 9 grams prot per 8 oz	6 oz	99	3.98	1.15	18.64	0	53	5	138	1	0.06	177
yogurt, fruit, lofat, 9 grams prot per 8 oz, fort w/ vitamin d	6 oz	99	3.98	1.15	18.64	0	53	5	138	52	0.06	177
yogurt, fruit, lofat, w/lo cal sweetener	6 oz	105	4.86	1.41	18.6	0	58	6	152	1	0.07	194
yogurt, fruit, lowfat, w/ lo cal swtnr, fort w/ vitamin d	6 oz	105	4.86	1.41	18.6	0	58	6	152	52	0.07	194
yogurt, frz, choc, non-fat milk, w/ lo cal swtnr	1 cup	107	4.4	0.8	19.7	2	81	4	159	0	0.04	339
yogurt, frz, flavors not choc, nonfat milk, w/ low-calorie swtnr	.5 cup	104	4.4	0.8	19.7	2	81	4	159	0	0.04	339
yogurt, frz, flavors other than choc, lowfat	7 oz	139	8	2.5	21	0	45	45	200	2	0	108
yogurt, greek, fruit, whl milk	7 oz	106	7.33	3	12.29	0	37	10	100	0	0	113
yogurt, greek, pln, lowfat	7 oz	73	9.95	1.92	3.94	0	34	10	115	0	0.04	141
yogurt, greek, pln, nonfat	5.3 oz	59	10.19	0.39	3.6	0	36	5	110	0	0.07	141
yogurt, greek, pln, whl milk	5.3 oz	97	9	5	3.98	0	35	13	100	0	0	141
yogurt, greek, strawberry, lowfat	5.3 oz	103	8.17	2.57	11.89	1	33	12	88	0	0.07	129
yogurt, greek, strawberry, nonfat	5.3 oz	82	8.05	0.15	12.07	0.6	33	4	97	40	0.09	132
yogurt, greek, vanilla, lowfat	5.3 oz	95	8.64	2.5	9.54	0	40	5	100	35	0.04	123
yogurt, greek, vanilla, nonfat	5.3 oz	78	8.64	0.18	10.37	0.5	34	3	99	35	0.04	123
yogurt, pln, lofat, 12 grams prot per 8 oz	6 oz	63	5.25	1.55	7.04	0	70	6	183	1	0.08	234
yogurt, pln, skim milk, 13 grams prot per 8 oz	6 oz	56	5.73	0.18	7.68	0	77	2	199	0	0.09	255
yogurt, pln, whl milk, 8 grams prot per 8 oz	6 oz	61	3.47	3.25	4.66	0	46	13	121	2	0.05	155
yogurt, van or lem flav, nonfat milk, swtnd w/low-calorie swtnr	6 oz	43	3.86	0.18	7.5	0	59	2	143	0	0.12	177
yogurt, van/lem flav, nonfat milk, w/ lo-cal swtnr, fort w/vit d	6 oz	43	3.86	0.18	7.5	0	59	2	143	47	0.12	177
yogurt, vanilla flavor, lowfat milk, swtnd w/ lo cal swtnr	6 oz	86	4.93	1.25	13.8	0	66	5	171	1	0.07	219
yogurt, vanilla, lofat, 11 grams prot per 8 oz	6 oz	85	4.93	1.25	13.8	0	66	5	171	1	0.07	219
yogurt, vanilla, lofat, 11 grams prot per 8 oz, fort w/ vit d	6 oz	85	4.93	1.25	13.8	0	66	5	171	47	0.07	219
yogurt, vanilla, non-fat	1 cup	78	2.94	0	17.04	0	47	3	118	35	0	141

From the USDA National Nutrient Database for Standard Reference, Release 28 (2015)

EXERCISE CHART

Estimated calories burned per hour based on body weight

Activity	130 lbs.	155 lbs.	190 lbs.
aerobics, general	354	422	518
aerobics, high impact	413	493	604
aerobics, low impact	295	352	431
archery (non-hunting)	207	246	302
automobile repair	177	211	259
backpacking, general	413	493	604
badminton, competitive	413	493	604
badminton, social, general	266	317	388
basketball, game	472	563	690
basketball, non-game, general	354	422	518
basketball, officiating	413	493	604
basketball, shooting baskets	266	317	388
basketball, wheelchair	384	457	561
bicycling, < 10 mph, leisure	236	281	345
bicycling, > 20 mph, racing	944	1,126	1,380
bicycling, 10-11.9 mph, light effort	354	422	518
bicycling, 12-13.9 mph, moderate effort	472	563	690
bicycling, 14-15.9 mph, vigorous effort	590	704	863
bicycling, 16-19 mph, very fast, racing	708	844	1035
bicycling, bmx or mountain	502	598	733
bicycling, stationary, general	295	352	431
bicycling, stationary, light effort	325	387	474
bicycling, stationary, moderate effort	413	493	604
bicycling, stationary, very light effort	177	211	259
bicycling, stationary, very vigorous effort	738	880	1,078
bicycling, stationary, vigorous effort	620	739	906
billiards	148	176	216

Activity	130 lbs.	155 lbs.	190 lbs.
bowling	177	211	259
boxing, in ring, general	708	844	1,035
boxing, punching bag	354	422	518
boxing, sparring	531	633	776
broomball	413	493	604
calisthenics (push-ups, sit-ups), vigorous effort	472	563	690
calisthenics, home, light/moderate effort	266	317	388
canoeing, on camping trip	236	281	345
canoeing, rowing, > 6 mph, vigorous effort	708	844	1,035
canoeing, rowing, crewing, competition	708	844	1,035
canoeing, rowing, light effort	177	211	259
canoeing, rowing, moderate effort	413	493	604
carpentry, general	207	246	302
carrying heavy loads, such as bricks	472	563	690
child care: sitting, kneeling, dressing, feeding	177	211	259
child care: standing-dressing, feeding	207	246	302
circuit training, general	472	563	690
cleaning, heavy, vigorous effort	266	317	388
cleaning, house, general	207	246	302
cleaning, light, moderate effort	148	176	216
coaching: football, soccer, basketball, etc.	236	281	345
construction, outside, remodeling	325	387	474
cooking or food preparation	148	176	216
cricket (batting, bowling)	295	352	431
croquet	148	176	216
curling	236	281	345
dancing, aerobic, ballet or modern, twist	354	422	518
dancing, ballroom, fast	325	387	474

Activity	130 lbs.	155 lbs.	190 lbs.
dancing, ballroom, slow	177	211	259
dancing, general	266	317	388
darts, wall or lawn	148	176	216
diving, springboard or platform	177	211	259
electrical work, plumbing	207	246	302
farming, baling hay, cleaning barn	472	563	690
farming, milking by hand	177	211	259
farming, shoveling grain	325	387	474
fencing	354	422	518
fishing from boat, sitting	148	176	216
fishing from river bank, standing	207	246	302
fishing in stream, in waders	354	422	518
fishing, general	236	281	345
fishing, ice, sitting	118	141	173
football or baseball, playing catch	148	176	216
football, competitive	531	633	776
football, touch, flag, general	472	563	690
frisbee playing, general	177	211	259
frisbee, ultimate	207	246	302
gardening, general	295	352	431
golf, carrying clubs	325	387	474
golf, general	236	281	345
golf, miniature or driving range	177	211	259
golf, pulling clubs	295	352	431
golf, using power cart	207	246	302
gymnastics, general	236	281	345
hacky sack	236	281	345
handball, general	708	844	1,035
handball, team	472	563	690

Activity	130 lbs.	155 lbs.	190 lbs.
hiking, cross country	354	422	518
hockey, field	472	563	690
hockey, ice	472	563	690
horse grooming	354	422	518
horse racing, galloping	472	563	690
horseback riding, general	236	281	345
horseback riding, trotting	384	457	561
horseback riding, walking	148	176	216
hunting, general	295	352	431
jai alai	708	844	1,035
jogging, general	413	493	604
judo, karate, kick boxing, tae kwan do	590	704	863
kayaking	295	352	431
kickball	413	493	604
lacrosse	472	563	690
marching band, playing instrument (walking)	236	281	345
marching, rapidly, military	384	457	561
motocross	236	281	345
moving furniture, household	354	422	518
moving household items, boxes, upstairs	531	633	776
moving household items, carrying boxes	413	493	604
mowing lawn, general	325	387	474
mowing lawn, riding mower	148	176	216
music playing, cello, flute, horn, woodwind	118	141	173
music playing, drums	236	281	345
music playing, guitar, classical, folk (sitting)	118	141	173
music playing, guitar, rock/roll band (standing)	177	211	259
music playing, piano, organ, violin, trumpet	148	176	216
paddleboat	236	281	345

Activity	130 lbs.	155 lbs.	190 lbs.
painting, papering, plastering, scraping	266	317	388
polo	472	563	690
pushing or pulling stroller with child	148	176	216
race walking	384	457	561
racquetball, casual, general	413	493	604
racquetball, competitive	590	704	863
raking lawn	236	281	345
rock climbing, ascending rock	649	774	949
rock climbing, rappelling	472	563	690
rope jumping, fast	708	844	1,035
rope jumping, moderate, general	590	704	863
rope jumping, slow	472	563	690
rowing, stationary, light effort	561	669	819
rowing, stationary, moderate effort	413	493	604
rowing, stationary, very vigorous effort	708	844	1035
rowing, stationary, vigorous effort	502	598	733
rugby	590	704	863
running, 10 mph (6-min. mile)	944	1,126	1,380
running, 10.9 mph (5.5-min. mile)	1,062	1,267	1,553
running, 5 mph (12-min. mile)	472	563	690
running, 5.2 mph (11.5-min. mile)	531	633	776
running, 6 mph (10-min. mile)	590	704	863
running, 6.7 mph (9-min. mile)	649	774	949
running, 7 mph (8.5-min. mile)	679	809	992
running, 7.5 mph (8-min. mile)	738	880	1,078
running, 8 mph (7.5-min. mile)	797	950	1,165
running, 8.6 mph (7-min. mile)	826	985	1,208
running, 9 mph (6.5-min. mile)	885	1,056	1,294

Activity	130 lbs.	155 lbs.	190 lbs.
running, cross country	531	633	776
running, general	472	563	690
running, in place	472	563	690
running, on a track, team practice	590	704	863
running, stairs, up	885	1,056	1,294
running, training, pushing wheelchair	472	563	690
running, wheeling, general	177	211	259
sailing, boat/board, windsurfing, general	177	211	259
sailing, in competition	295	352	431
scrubbing floors, on hands and knees	325	387	474
shoveling snow, by hand	354	422	518
shuffleboard, lawn bowling	177	211	259
sitting-playing with children, light effort	148	176	216
skateboarding	295	352	431
skating, ice, 9 mph or less	325	387	474
skating, ice, general	413	493	604
skating, ice, rapidly, > 9 mph	531	633	776
skating, ice, speed, competitive	885	1,056	1,294
skating, roller	413	493	604
ski jumping (climb up carrying skis)	413	493	604
ski machine, general	561	669	819
skiing, cross-country, > 8.0 mph, racing	826	985	1,208
skiing, cross-country, moderate effort	472	563	690
skiing, cross-country, slow or light effort	413	493	604
skiing, cross-country, uphill, maximum effort	974	1,161	1,423
skiing, cross-country, vigorous effort	531	633	776
skiing, downhill, light effort	295	352	431
skiing, downhill, moderate effort	354	422	518

Activity	130 lbs.	155 lbs.	190 lbs.
skiing, downhill, vigorous effort, racing	472	563	690
skiing, snow, general	413	493	604
skiing, water	354	422	518
ski-mobiling, water	413	493	604
skin diving, scuba diving, general	413	493	604
sledding, tobogganing, bobsledding, luge	413	493	604
snorkeling	295	352	431
snowshoeing	472	563	690
snowmobiling	207	246	302
soccer, casual, general	413	493	604
soccer, competitive	590	704	863
softball or baseball, fast or slow pitch	295	352	431
softball, officiating	354	422	518
squash	708	844	1,035
stair-treadmill ergometer, general	354	422	518
standing-packing/unpacking boxes	207	246	302
stretching, hatha yoga	236	281	345
surfing, body or board	177	211	259
sweeping garage, sidewalk	236	281	345
swimming laps, freestyle, fast, vigorous effort	590	704	863
swimming laps, freestyle, light/moderate effort	472	563	690
swimming, backstroke, general	472	563	690
swimming, breaststroke, general	590	704	863
swimming, butterfly, general	649	774	949
swimming, leisurely, general	354	422	518
swimming, sidestroke, general	472	563	690
swimming, synchronized	472	563	690
swimming, treading water, fast/vigorous	590	704	863

Activity	130 lbs.	155 lbs.	190 lbs.
swimming, treading water, moderate effort	236	281	345
table tennis, ping pong	236	281	345
tai chi	236	281	345
teaching aerobics class	354	422	518
tennis, doubles	354	422	518
tennis, general	413	493	604
tennis, singles	472	563	690
unicycling	295	352	431
volleyball, beach	472	563	690
volleyball, competitive, in gymnasium	236	281	345
volleyball, noncompetitive; 6 to 9 member team	177	211	259
walk/run-playing with children-moderate	236	281	345
walk/run-playing with children-vigorous	295	352	431
walking, 2 mph, slow pace	148	176	216
walking, 3 mph, moderate pace, walking dog	207	246	302
walking, 3.5 mph, uphill	354	422	518
walking, 4 mph, very brisk pace	236	281	345
walking, carrying infant or 15-lb. load	207	246	302
walking, grass track	295	352	431
walking, upstairs	472	563	690
walking, using crutches	236	281	345
wallyball, general	413	493	604
water aerobics, water calisthenics	236	281	345
water polo	590	704	863
water volleyball	177	211	259
weight lifting or body building, vigorous effort	354	422	518
weight lifting, light or moderate effort	177	211	259
whitewater rafting, kayaking, or canoeing	295	352	431

From the State of Wisconsin, Department of Health and Family Services, Division of Public Health, PPH 40109 (09/05)

Sources for Essential Vitamins & Minerals

CALCIUM Food	Portion Size	Calcium (mg) in Standard Portion
pasteurized processed American cheese	2 ounces	593
Parmesan cheese, hard	1½ ounces	503
plain yogurt, nonfat	8 ounces	452
Romano cheese	1½ ounces	452
almond milk (all flavors)	1 cup	451
pasteurized processed Swiss cheese	2 ounces	438
tofu, raw, regular, with calcium sulfate	½ cup	434
Gruyère cheese	1½ ounces	430
plain yogurt, low-fat	8 ounces	415

VITAMIN D Food	Portion Size	Vitamin D (µg) in Standard Portion
salmon, sockeye, canned	3 ounces	17.9
trout, rainbow, farmed, cooked	3 ounces	16.2
salmon, chinook, smoked	3 ounces	14.5
swordfish, cooked	3 ounces	14.1
salmon, pink, canned	3 ounces	12.3
fish oil, cod liver	1 teaspoon	11.3
salmon, sockeye, cooked	3 ounces	11.1
salmon, pink, cooked	3 ounces	11.1
mushrooms, portabella, exposed to UV light, grilled	½ cup	7.9

From the USDA Dietary Guidelines for Americans, 2015–2020

IRON Food	Portion Size	Iron (mg) in Standard Portion
shellfish, cooked	3 ounces	28
beef liver, cooked	3½ ounces	6.5
pumpkin seeds	1 ounce	4.2
spinach	3½ ounces	3.6
tofu, raw, regular	½ cup	3.6
lentils, cooked	½ cup	3.3
dark chocolate	1 ounce	3.3
quinoa, cooked	1 cup	2.8
red meat, cooked	3½ ounces	2.7

POTASSIUM Food	Portion Size	Potassium (mg) in Standard Portion
potato, baked, flesh & skin	1 medium	941
prune juice, canned	1 cup	707
carrot juice, canned	1 cup	689
passion fruit juice, yellow or purple	1 cup	687
tomato paste, canned	¼ cup	669
beet greens, cooked from fresh	½ cup	654
azuki beans, cooked	½ cup	612
white beans, canned	½ cup	595
plain yogurt, nonfat	1 cup	579

FIBER Food	Portion Size	Dietary Fiber (g) in Standard Portion
high-fiber bran ready-to-eat cereal	½–¾ cup	9.1-14.3
navy beans, cooked	½ cup	9.6
small white beans, cooked	½ cup	9.3
yellow beans, cooked	½ cup	9.2
shredded wheat ready-to-eat cereal	1–1¼ cups	5.0-9.0
cranberry (roman) beans, cooked	½ cup	8.9
azuki beans, cooked	½ cup	8.4
French beans, cooked	½ cup	8.3
split peas, cooked	½ cup	8.1

Before

[front]

[side]